FERTILITY DIET COOKBOOK FOR WOMEN

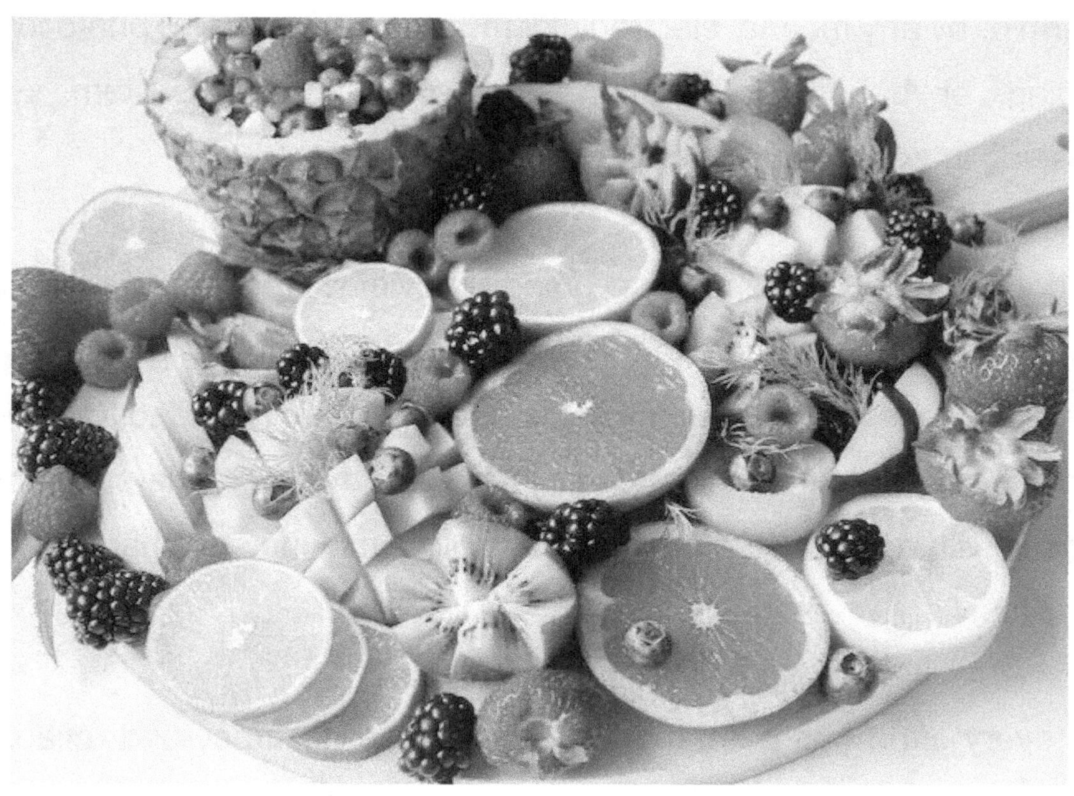

Mouth-watering Recipes for Women on their Journey to Motherhood

SHEBA YOHANNA

Table of content

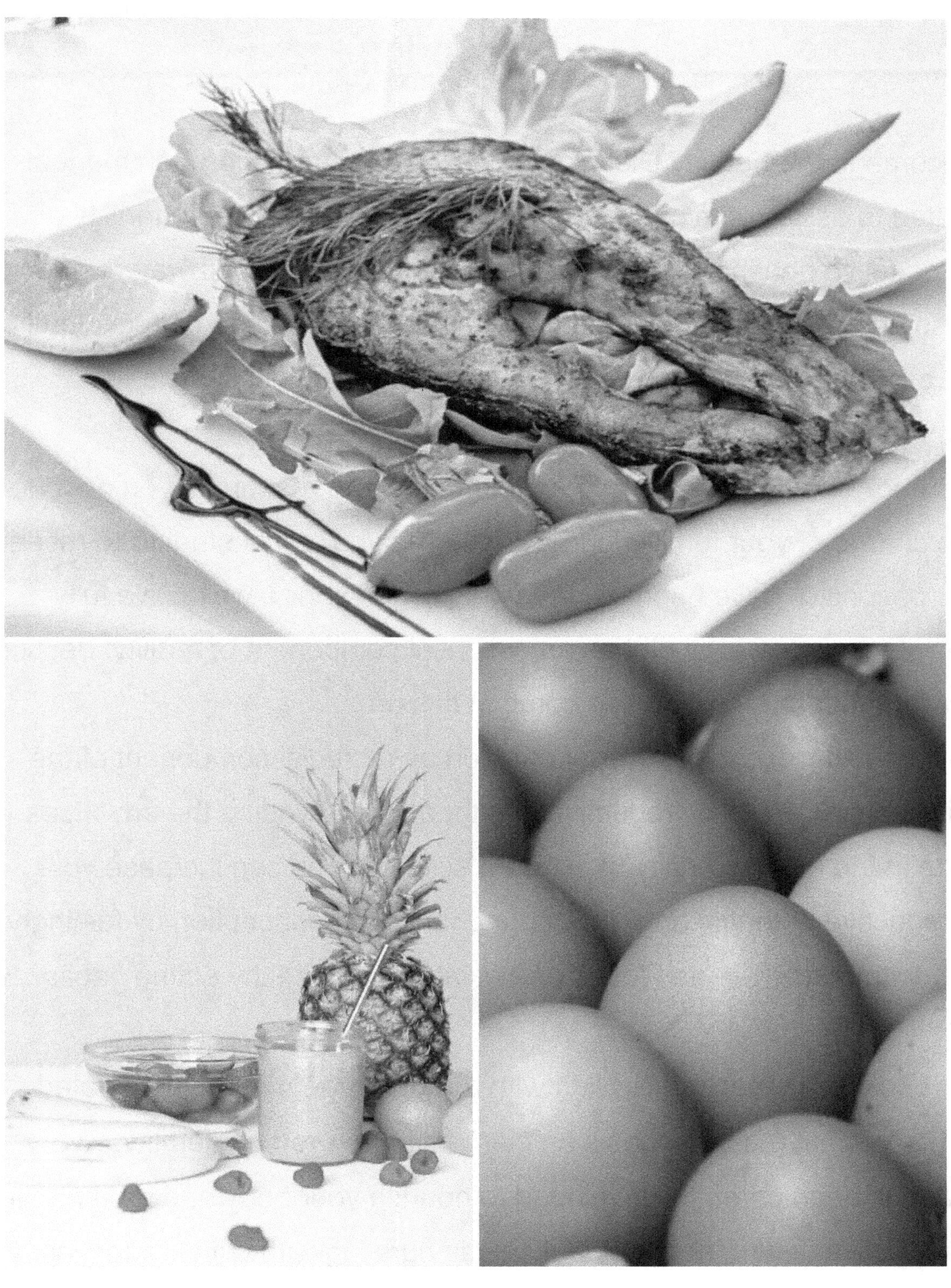

Introduction

Welcome to the Fertility Diet Cookbook, a useful and thorough manual created to assist women in achieving their goals of optimum fertility and reproductive health. This book offers more than just mouthwatering recipes; it also acts as a roadmap for comprehending how nutrition affects fertility and offers insightful advice on how to lead a balanced lifestyle that supports a healthy reproductive system.

This book strives to give you the information and resources you need to take charge of your fertility journey, whether you're just starting to research your options or have been trying to get pregnant for a while. We fully believe in the power of diet as an essential component of fertility, despite how far modern medicine has come in this area.

We fully believe in the power of nutrition as a crucial component of the holistic approach to reproductive health, notwithstanding the advances made in the field of fertility by modern science. You can increase your reproductive potential and raise your chances of conception by fueling your body with nutrient-dense foods and establishing healthy eating habits.

This cookbook's pages are filled with a wide range of expertly created dishes that have an emphasis on elements that promote fertility. Every meal has been carefully developed to nourish your body and promote your reproductive health, from colorful salads bursting with critical vitamins and minerals to energetic smoothies filled with antioxidants to hearty entrees fortified with fertility-enhancing elements.

Beyond the recipes, we explore the critical facets of nutrition and provide evidence-based guidance to assist you in making decisions about your diet. We go into detail about the essential nutrients that are vital to fertility and the best places to get them, making it easier for you to understand how to use them in delicious and practical ways in your meals. Along with nutrition, we also look at how lifestyle factors like stress management, exercise, and sleep affect fertility. This will help you design a well-rounded strategy to maximize your fertility potential.

While the process of becoming pregnant can be complicated and intensely personal, we hope that this cookbook can serve as an educational and empowering tool for you. We sincerely think that by taking control of your nutrition and embracing the knowledge of a diet designed specifically for fertility, you may dramatically increase your chances of becoming pregnant and prepare the road for a safe pregnancy.

We are aware of the challenges, doubts, and feelings that can accompany the fertility journey, and we hope that this book will help you achieve your goal of parenthood as well as serve as a reliable guide as you work toward becoming a healthier, more vibrant version of yourself.

Remember that the goal here is to nurture your body, adopt a good outlook, and recognize the incredible potential you possess. This is not just about recipes. Welcome to the Fertility Diet Cookbook. We're here to support you along the road by providing inspiration, knowledge, and empowerment.

Chapter 1: Understanding Female Fertility

Understanding female fertility entails learning about the reproductive system and the elements that influence a woman's ability to conceive. It is essential for both men and women who want to start a family or individuals who simply want to better understand their bodies.

Female fertility is mostly dependent on the menstrual cycle, which is controlled by several hormonal changes in a woman's body. The cycle usually lasts about 28 days, but this can vary from person to person. During this cycle, an egg is released from one of the ovaries and travels down the fallopian tubes, where it can be fertilized by sperm. If fertilization does not occur, the uterine lining is lost during menstruation.

While fertility is strongest around the time of ovulation, which normally happens around mid-cycle, women can conceive at any time during their menstrual cycle. Sperm can live for several days inside a woman's reproductive system, boosting the chances of fertilization if intercourse occurs a few days before ovulation.

Age, underlying health issues, hormone imbalances, weight, and lifestyle choices can all have an impact on female fertility. Women's fertility normally declines as they age, and the chance of difficulties during pregnancy rises.

Understanding the signs and symptoms of ovulation might aid in determining the most fertile days. Changes in cervical mucus consistency, a minor elevation in basal body temperature, and mild soreness on one side of the pelvis are examples. However, it is critical to check with a healthcare practitioner for a more precise assessment of fertility and any potential issues.

Overall, understanding female fertility helps women to make informed decisions about family planning and reproductive health. It helps people understand their physiology and lays the groundwork for a healthy and joyful reproductive journey.

The Science Behind Female Fertility

The fascinating subject of female fertility involves a complicated interplay of biological mechanisms. Female fertility can be summed up as a woman's capacity to conceive and give birth to children. This amazing occurrence is made possible by several complex regulatory processes that are under the control of the female reproductive system.

The ovulation process is one of the most important aspects of female fertility. A mature egg is released from the ovary during ovulation. In most women of reproductive age, it is a monthly cyclical occurrence. A spike in luteinizing hormone (LH), which is managed by the brain's hypothalamus and pituitary gland, causes the egg to release.

Once released, the egg moves via the fallopian tubes in the direction of the uterus. It may be fertilized by sperm during this travel, which would result in pregnancy. Unfertilized eggs are discharged through menstruation if fertilization is unsuccessful.

Female fertility is influenced by several additional factors in addition to ovulation. These consist of the well-being and caliber of the eggs, the state of the reproductive system as a whole, the hormonal balance, and the existence of any underlying medical disorders.

Age is a significant factor in female fertility as well. The quantity and caliber of eggs that remain in the ovaries as women get older is known as their ovarian reserve. The odds of becoming pregnant for women over the age of 40 significantly diminish due to this natural decline in fertility.

It's important to note that a variety of conditions, including hormonal imbalances, PCOS, endometriosis, and particular lifestyle decisions like smoking, binge drinking, and eating poorly, can impair female fertility. These factors can have different effects on different women, and addressing them may call for medical intervention or a change in their way of living.

Last but not least, improvements in reproductive medicine have given women choices to improve their odds of getting pregnant. In vitro fertilization (IVF) and fertility preservation techniques have created new opportunities and given women more control over their reproductive decisions.

Women can be empowered to make knowledgeable choices about their reproductive health by understanding the facts underpinning female fertility. Additionally, it emphasizes the importance of routine checkups, leading a healthy lifestyle, and offering supporting healthcare services to women who might have trouble getting pregnant.

The ability of a woman to conceive and carry a pregnancy to term is determined by a variety of circumstances. The following are some significant variables that may affect female fertility:

- **Age:** One of the biggest influences on a woman's fertility is her age. The amount and quality of a woman's eggs deteriorate with age because she has a limited number of eggs when she is born.
- **Hormonal Balance:** When a woman's ovulation is inconsistent or nonexistent, it might be challenging for her to get pregnant. The balance of hormones can be disturbed by conditions like thyroid problems or polycystic ovarian syndrome (PCOS).
- **Ovulation Disorders:** Obstacles to the release of eggs from the ovaries for fertilization, such as blocked fallopian tubes, can cause issues with ovulation.
- **Structural Issues:** Abnormalities in the reproductive organs, such as uterine fibroids or aberrant uterine shape (e.g., septum, double uterus), might impact fertility.
- **Reproductive Infections:** Certain infections, such as sexually transmitted infections (STIs), can cause scarring or damage to the fallopian tubes or uterus, leading to infertility.
- **Medical Conditions:** Chronic conditions such as diabetes, autoimmune disorders, or some cancers might influence fertility due to their effect on reproductive organs or hormonal balance.

- **Lifestyle Factors:** Certain lifestyle choices, such as smoking, excessive alcohol consumption, drug use, and obesity, can lower conception rates in women.
- **Stress:** Prolonged mental or physical stress can disrupt the menstrual cycle and cause ovulation problems.
- **Genetic Factors:** Some genetic diseases acquired from parents, such as Turner syndrome or Fragile X syndrome, might impact fertility.

It's crucial to remember that each woman's fertility is unique, and the factors that influence fertility might differ from person to person. A more personalized evaluation and help with fertility concerns might be obtained by consulting a healthcare expert.

Hormonal Balance and its Impact on Fertility

Hormonal balance is important for our overall health, but it is even more important when it comes to fertility. To regulate the reproductive system and maintain appropriate functioning, our bodies rely on a complicated interaction of hormones.

A hormonal imbalance can be defined as an excess or lack of specific hormones, which disrupts the delicate balance and, as a result, affects fertility. Hormonal abnormalities can affect both men and women, resulting in a variety of reproductive difficulties.

In women, hormonal imbalances can notably impact the menstrual cycle, ovulation, and the ability to conceive. Conditions such as polycystic ovary syndrome (PCOS) often result in irregular periods and anovulation (lack of ovulation), making it challenging to get pregnant. In addition, high levels of certain hormones, such as prolactin or luteinizing hormone (LH), can also interfere with ovulation and fertility. Men's fertility can also be strongly influenced by hormone imbalances. Low testosterone levels, for example, can affect sperm production, reduce the quality and quantity of sperm, and ultimately impact fertility. Elevated levels of follicle-stimulating hormone (FSH) may indicate underlying issues with the testicles, resulting in decreased sperm production and fertility.

It is crucial to strike a balance when it comes to our hormones. Fortunately, there are various ways to restore hormonal balance and support fertility. Lifestyle modifications, including regular exercise, a balanced diet, stress reduction, and adequate sleep, can positively impact hormonal levels. Furthermore, certain medications or hormone therapies may be prescribed by healthcare professionals to restore balance in specific cases. Understanding our bodies and their hormonal patterns is vital when it comes to fertility. Seeking medical advice from a reproductive specialist can provide valuable insights and guidance throughout the fertility journey. Hormonal balance is a key factor to consider, and by addressing any imbalances, both men and women can optimize their chances of conceiving and achieving their family goals.

Exploring the Menstrual Cycle and Ovulation

Ovulation and the menstrual cycle are fascinating components of a woman's reproductive system. The monthly set of changes that occur in a woman's body to prepare for pregnancy is referred to as the menstrual cycle. It usually lasts around 28 days, however, this varies from person to person.

Menstruation is the first stage of the menstrual cycle, and it involves the loss of the thicker uterine lining. When an egg discharged during the previous cycle was not fertilized, this occurs. Menstruation typically lasts 3-7 days and is associated with varied degrees of discomfort and hormonal changes.

The body starts the follicular phase following menstruation. Follicle-stimulating hormone (FSH) from the pituitary gland stimulates the ovaries to generate many follicles during this period. Each follicle contains an immature egg, which produces estrogen as it develops. This rise in estrogen causes the uterine lining to thicken in preparation for a possible pregnancy.

A spike of luteinizing hormone (LH) is released in the middle of the cycle, causing one dominant follicle to deliver a mature egg. This is known as ovulation, and it normally occurs around day 14 of a 28-day cycle. Ovulation is the most fertile phase of the menstrual cycle, and it is during this period that the egg can be fertilized by sperm if intercourse happens.

The body enters the luteal phase after ovulation. The burst follicle, now known as the corpus luteum, generates progesterone, which aids in the preservation of the uterine lining during pregnancy. If there is no fertilization, the corpus luteum degenerates, progesterone levels fall, and the menstrual cycle begins anew with menstruation.

Understanding one's menstrual cycle and ovulation can be beneficial for many reasons, including family planning, fertility awareness, and understanding hormonal changes that frequently accompany various physical and mental symptoms that some women experience throughout their cycle.

It's important to remember that each woman's menstrual cycle is unique and might vary in length, regularity, and symptoms. Tracking patterns and symptoms can be beneficial for people who want to better understand their bodies or manage their reproductive health.

Lifestyle and Environmental Factors Affecting Fertility

Fertility can be greatly influenced by lifestyle and environmental variables. Our reproductive health can be influenced by the decisions we make and the circumstances in which we live. Here are a few things to think about:

- **Diet and Nutrition:** Eating a well-balanced diet and getting enough nutrients can help with hormonal balance and reproductive function. Fertility can benefit from a diet rich in fruits, vegetables, whole grains, lean proteins, and healthy fats.

- **Weight and Exercise:** Excessive body weight and underweight can both affect hormone function, resulting in irregular menstrual cycles and diminished fertility. Regular exercise and maintaining a healthy weight can help with fertility.

- **Substance Abuse and Smoking:** Smoking cigarettes and using recreational drugs such as marijuana can hurt fertility in both men and women. These drugs can lower sperm count and motility in men while interfering with ovulation and increasing the chance of ectopic pregnancies in women.

- **Alcohol Use:** Heavy alcohol use has been associated with lower fertility in both men and women. It can interfere with hormone production, sperm quality, and ovulation.

- **Stress and Mental Health:** Excessive stress can impair fertility by interfering with natural hormonal balance and menstrual cycles. Stress-reduction measures such as exercise, meditation, or therapy can be beneficial.

- **Environmental Factors:** Certain chemicals and pollutants in our environment can have an impact on fertility. Pesticides, pollutants, and chemicals found in plastics and personal care items are examples of these. It is critical to be aware of these factors and to limit your exposure wherever feasible.

- **Age:** For both men and women, age is an important determinant of fertility. Women's fertility begins to wane in their late twenties and declines dramatically after the age of 35. Men's fertility may fall with age as well, with a steady decrease in sperm quality and production.

Individuals and couples can improve their chances of conceiving by understanding and addressing certain lifestyle and environmental factors. Consultation with healthcare professionals, such as fertility specialists, can provide extra assistance that is targeted to unique situations and medical conditions.

Chapter 2: The Foundation of a Fertility-Friendly Diet

A fertility-friendly diet is built on nutrient-dense foods that promote reproductive health and hormonal balance. It contains healthful grains, fruits and vegetables, lean proteins, healthy fats, and dairy or dairy substitutes. These foods provide vitamins, minerals, antioxidants, and phytochemicals that are necessary for healthy fertility.

Whole grains, such as quinoa and brown rice, are high in fiber, which benefits blood sugar regulation and hormone balance. Fruits and vegetables are high in vitamins and antioxidants, which help to produce healthy eggs and sperm. Because of their high folate concentration, leafy greens like spinach and kale are especially advantageous for fetal growth.

Lean proteins, such as fish, chicken, and lentils, are high in protein but low in saturated fat. They supply vital amino acids that aid in reproductive health. Healthy fats found in avocados, olive oil, and nuts are essential for hormone production and function. Omega-3 fatty acids, which are abundant in fatty fish such as salmon, are especially favorable to reproductive health.

Calcium-rich meals, such as dairy products or dairy alternatives such as almond milk or soy milk, boost the overall reproductive system and aid in the formation of healthy eggs and sperm.

Aside from these basic foods, it's critical to stay hydrated and minimize your intake of processed meals, trans fats, and sugar. Regular physical activity and stress-reduction approaches such as meditation or yoga can supplement the benefits of a fertility-friendly diet. For individualized nutritional suggestions and counseling, it is also advisable to consult with a healthcare practitioner or a licensed dietitian.

The Role of Nutrition in Promoting Female Fertility

Proper nutrition is critical in maintaining an individual's overall health and well-being, and this is especially true for women. A woman's diet is critical at all stages of her life, from childhood through adolescence, pregnancy to lactation, and throughout her adult years.

Maintaining a well-balanced diet rich in vitamins, minerals, proteins, carbs, and healthy fats is an important element of female nutrition. This is crucial to guarantee that the body receives all of the necessary nutrients for physical and mental growth, development, and maintenance. Adequate nutrition promotes a healthy body weight, a strong immune system, a lower risk of chronic diseases, and energy for everyday activities.

In terms of specific dietary demands, women often require more important nutrients than men. Iron, calcium, vitamin D, and folic acid are examples. Iron is essential for maintaining appropriate hemoglobin levels in the blood and preventing anemia, particularly during menstruation. Calcium and vitamin D are necessary for bone strength and health, preventing disorders such as osteoporosis. Folic acid is essential for pregnant women because it aids in the prevention of birth abnormalities of the brain and spine in growing embryos.

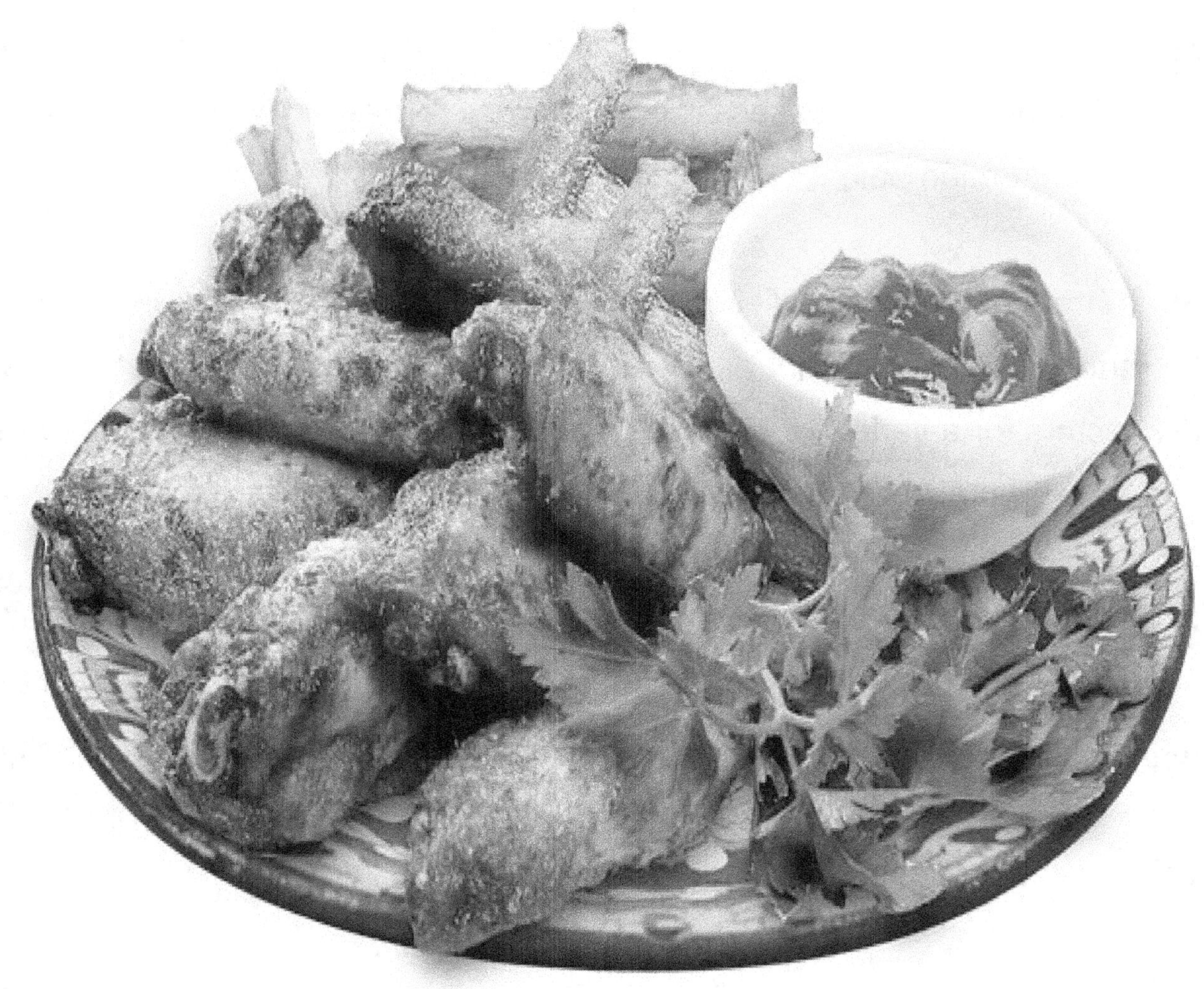

Female nutrition also includes the treatment of hormonal changes that occur during a woman's life. During menstruation, for example, the body requires adequate vitamins and minerals to restore lost blood and control hormonal changes. Furthermore, a woman's nutritional demands rise dramatically during pregnancy and breastfeeding to support the growth and development of the fetus or the nutritional needs of the newborn.

Nutrition can also play an important role in the management of certain health disorders that are more common in women. For example, eating omega-3-rich foods like fish, avocados, and walnuts can help lower inflammation and control symptoms of illnesses including polycystic ovarian syndrome (PCOS) and menstruation pain.

Furthermore, a balanced diet can aid in the maintenance of a healthy weight by reducing excess weight gain and obesity, both of which are established risk factors for a variety of diseases such as heart disease, type 2 diabetes, and several malignancies. Nutritional health also promotes good skin, hair, and nails, which improves the overall look and boosts self-esteem.
In addition to eating, women should engage in regular physical exercise to supplement their nutrition and maintain optimal health. Exercise aids in the maintenance of a healthy weight, the development of strong bones, the prevention of chronic diseases, the improvement of mental health, and the enhancement of general well-being.

To summarize, diet plays a critical role in improving female health and well-being. Women may give their bodies the critical nutrients they require for growth, development, and maintenance by eating a nutritious and well-balanced diet. A good diet is essential for keeping a healthy body weight, boosting the immune system, and lowering the risk of chronic illnesses, all of which lead to a happier and better life.

Key Nutrients for Optimal Reproductive Health

Individuals who want to start a family or just maintain a healthy reproductive system must have optimal reproductive health. While other critical nutrients help support and improve reproductive health, the following stand out:

- **Folic acid,** often known as vitamin B9, is necessary for both men and women. It is essential for the production of DNA and the proper growth of a baby during pregnancy because it plays a critical function in tissue growth and cell development. Folic acid supplementation can also help lessen the chance of certain birth abnormalities.

- **Zinc:** Zinc is a vital nutrient for male reproductive health. It is essential for sperm generation, testosterone production, and general reproductive function. Men with low zinc levels are frequently infertile. Zinc-rich foods such as oysters, steak, pumpkin seeds, and legumes can help men maintain normal reproductive health.

- **Omega-3 Fatty Acids:** Omega-3 fatty acids, particularly EPA and DHA, are essential for hormonal balance, sperm production, and general reproductive health. Include fatty fish such as salmon, sardines, and mackerel in your diet, as well as walnuts, chia seeds, and flaxseeds, to ensure an appropriate intake of these critical nutrients.

- **Iron:** Iron is essential for the reproductive health of both men and women. It aids in the transportation of oxygen to the reproductive organs of women, promoting a healthy menstrual cycle and fertility. Iron aids in the generation of healthy sperm in men. It aids in the transportation of oxygen to the reproductive organs of women, promoting a healthy menstrual cycle and fertility. Iron aids in the generation of healthy sperm in men. Iron-rich meals such as lean meats, spinach, lentils, and fortified cereals can help keep iron levels optimal.

- **Vitamin C:** Vitamin C is an antioxidant that can improve sperm quality and defend against oxidative stress. This vital nutrient can be obtained by eating citrus fruits, berries, peppers, and leafy greens.

- **Vitamin E:** Vitamin E is another antioxidant that helps to keep reproductive organs healthy and protects sperm and egg cells from harm. Vitamin E can be found in nuts, seeds, sunflower oil, and spinach.

A well-balanced diet rich in fruits, vegetables, whole grains, lean proteins, and healthy fats is important for general reproductive health. Remember to remain hydrated, exercise regularly, manage stress, and avoid excessive alcohol and smoking, as these can have productive health.

Designing a Well-Balanced Fertility Diet

When creating a well-balanced fertility diet, it's critical to prioritize nutrient-rich foods that promote reproductive health. While there is no magical food that ensures conception, eating a well-balanced diet can help you get pregnant. Here are some important factors to consider:

1. Healthy Fats: Include unsaturated fat sources like avocados, nuts, seeds, and oily fish like salmon. These can help in hormone synthesis and nutrient absorption.

2. Plant Proteins: Choose protein sources that are plant-based, such as lentils, beans, quinoa, and tofu. They are high in fiber, vitamins, and minerals, and they can help with ovulation and hormone balance.

3. Complex Carbohydrates: Whole grains like brown rice, oats, and whole wheat bread are high in fiber and help balance blood sugar levels. High-refined carbs and sugars should be avoided because they can contribute to insulin resistance.

4. Colorful fruits and veggies: Include a variety of fruits and veggies on your plate because they are high in antioxidants, vitamins, and minerals that promote reproductive health. Dark leafy greens, citrus fruits, berries, and cruciferous vegetables such as broccoli and cauliflower are all high in antioxidants.

5. Iron-rich foods: Iron-rich foods include lean meat, poultry, seafood, spinach, and lentils. Iron promotes proper ovulation and aids in the transfer of oxygen to the reproductive organs.

6. Vitamin D: Spend time outside to help your body manufacture vitamin D naturally, or explore dietary sources such as fatty fish, egg yolks, fortified dairy, or plant-based milk. Vitamin D is essential for conception.

7. Antioxidant-Rich Foods: Increase your intake of berries, pomegranates, green tea, leafy greens, and nuts. Antioxidants shield eggs and sperm from the damaging effects of free radicals.

8. Hydration: Drink plenty of water to stay hydrated. It promotes healthy cervical mucus consistency and general body function.

9. Limit caffeine and alcohol intake: Both caffeine and alcohol can have negative effects on fertility, so it's best to consume them in moderation or avoid them altogether.

10. Individualization: Because everyone's body is different, it's critical to engage with a healthcare practitioner or nutritionist to adapt a fertility diet to your personal needs.

Maintaining a healthy lifestyle, controlling stress, getting regular exercise, and getting enough sleep are all crucial elements to consider when trying to conceive.

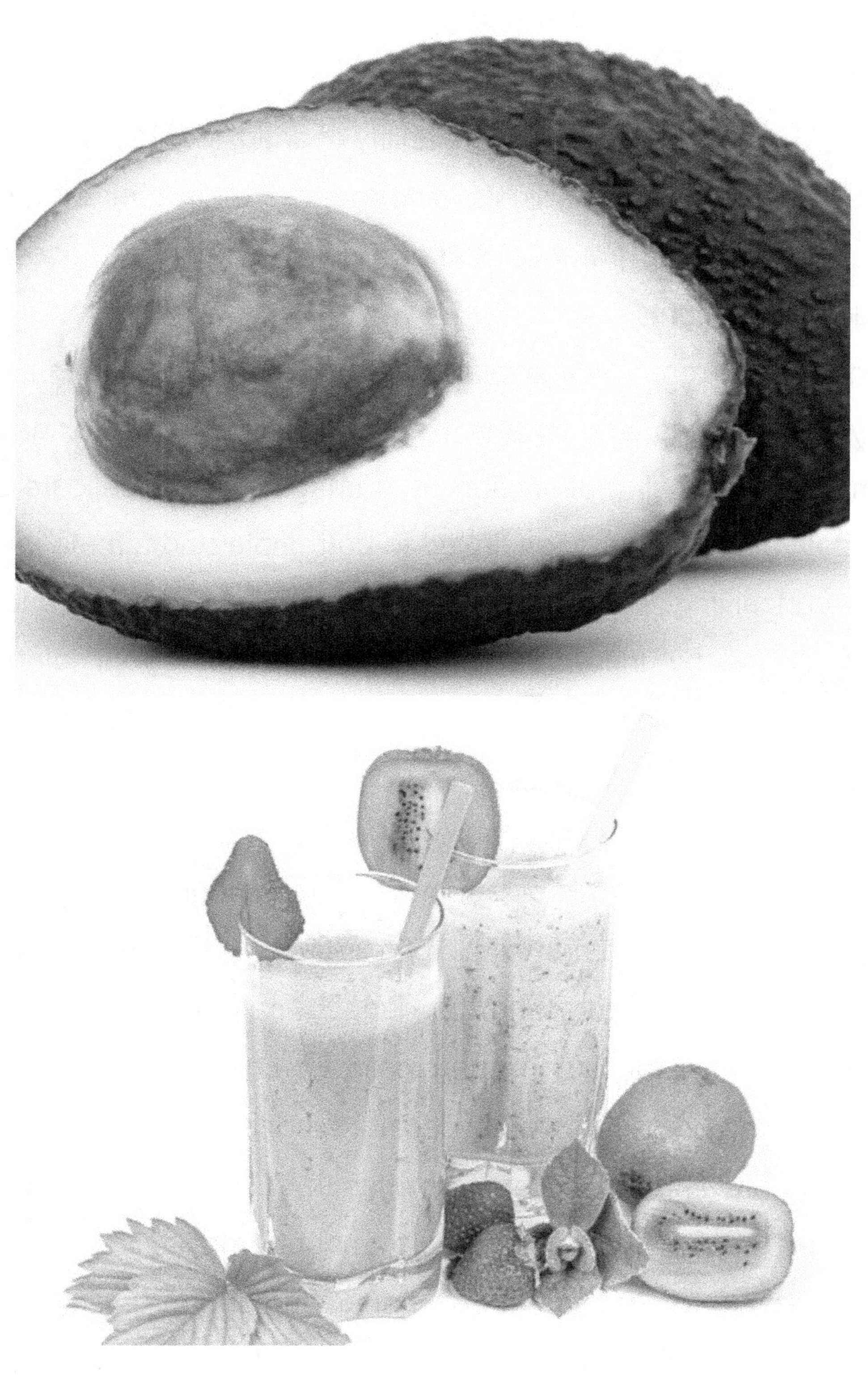

The Power of Antioxidants in Enhancing Fertility

Antioxidants have long been lauded for their health advantages, and their impact on fertility is no different. The ability of antioxidants to battle damaging chemicals known as free radicals is what gives them their strength. These free radicals have the potential to harm cells, especially those involved in reproductive function.

Male and female reproductive systems both rely on the health and function of many cells, tissues, and organs. Free radicals can cause oxidative stress, inflammation, and cell malfunction by damaging these delicate structures. This oxidative stress has been linked to both male and female infertility and difficulty conceiving. You can help neutralize free radicals and minimize oxidative stress by incorporating antioxidants into your diet or taking supplements. This can have a good effect on fertility and boost your chances of conceiving.

For women, antioxidants can improve fertility by protecting the health and quality of eggs, also known as oocytes. The amount and quality of eggs naturally decrease as women age. Antioxidants, on the other hand, can help minimize this loss by protecting the genetic material within the eggs from harm. Furthermore, antioxidants can maintain a healthy uterine environment for implantation and assist in a successful pregnancy.

Antioxidants are important for sperm health in men. Oxidative stress can have a deleterious impact on sperm count, motility, and morphology. Antioxidants help to fight this stress, enhancing sperm quality overall. This, in turn, improves fertility and raises the likelihood of a successful pregnancy.

It is crucial to remember that, while antioxidants can help with conception, they are not a cure-all for infertility. If you are having difficulty conceiving, you should consult with a healthcare provider or a fertility specialist. They can give you personalized counsel and recommendations based on your specific situation.

Including fruits, veggies, whole grains, and legumes in your diet is a fantastic method to organically improve your antioxidant consumption. Vitamin C, vitamin E, selenium, and zinc are among the primary antioxidants linked to increased fertility. Citrus fruits, berries, nuts, seeds, leafy greens, and entire grains contain them.

Maintaining a healthy lifestyle, including regular exercise, adequate relaxation, and stress management, is critical in promoting fertility. Antioxidants supplement these lifestyle factors by improving reproductive health and overall well-being.

Developing Healthy Eating Habits for Improved Fertility

Developing healthy eating habits is critical for overall well-being, and it can also play an important part in fertility improvement. A nutritious diet rich in fruits and vegetables can improve reproductive health, boost the chances of conception, and support a healthy pregnancy. Here are some suggestions for developing healthy eating habits for increased fertility:

- **Emphasize Whole Foods:** Include a variety of whole foods in your diet, such as fruits, vegetables, whole grains, lean meats, and healthy fats. Choose fresh, unprocessed foods high in important nutrients, vitamins, and minerals.

- **Consume antioxidant-rich foods:** Antioxidants assist in counteracting the effects of oxidative stress, which can impair fertility. Include antioxidant-rich foods in your regular diet, such as berries, leafy greens, nuts, seeds, and colorful fruits and vegetables.

- **Make Healthy Fats a Priority:** Healthy fats, particularly monounsaturated fats, and omega-3 fatty acids, are essential for hormonal balance and reproductive health. To ensure an appropriate amount of healthy fats, include avocados, nuts, seeds, olive oil, and fatty seafood in your diet.

- **Eat More Plant-Based Proteins:** Plant-based proteins such as beans, lentils, tofu, and quinoa can be high in protein while being low in saturated fat when compared to animal proteins. Choose these options more often to support reproductive health.

- **Stay Hydrated:** Water is necessary for overall health, including reproductive health. Drink plenty of water throughout the day to stay hydrated. Sugary beverages should be avoided in excess since they can hurt fertility.

- **Limit Processed Meals:** Processed meals are abundant in harmful fats, added sugars, and unnatural additives, all of which can harm fertility. Reduce your intake in favor of entire, nutrient-dense foods.

- **Caffeine and Alcohol Consumption in Moderation:** While there is no definitive consensus on the effects of caffeine and alcohol on fertility, it is best to consume them in moderation. Caffeine and alcohol use may interfere with hormone synthesis and fertility.

- **Practice Portion Control:** Maintain a healthy weight by paying attention to portion sizes, as both overweight and underweight disorders can interfere with fertility. Consult a qualified dietitian or nutritionist for assistance in determining the proper meal sizes for your unique needs.

- **Take a multivitamin:** While eating a well-balanced diet is the best way to get nutrients, taking a prenatal or multivitamin with critical nutrients like folate, iron, and vitamin D can help address nutritional gaps in your diet.

- **Seek practitioner advice:** Because each individual and couple is unique, it is best to speak with a healthcare practitioner or a registered dietitian who can provide individualized nutrition and reproductive advice.

Remember that building healthy eating habits for enhanced fertility requires time and persistence. Begin by adopting small, lasting dietary modifications and celebrate each step toward healthy living. You may improve your fertility and boost your chances of conceiving by fueling your body with nutritious foods.

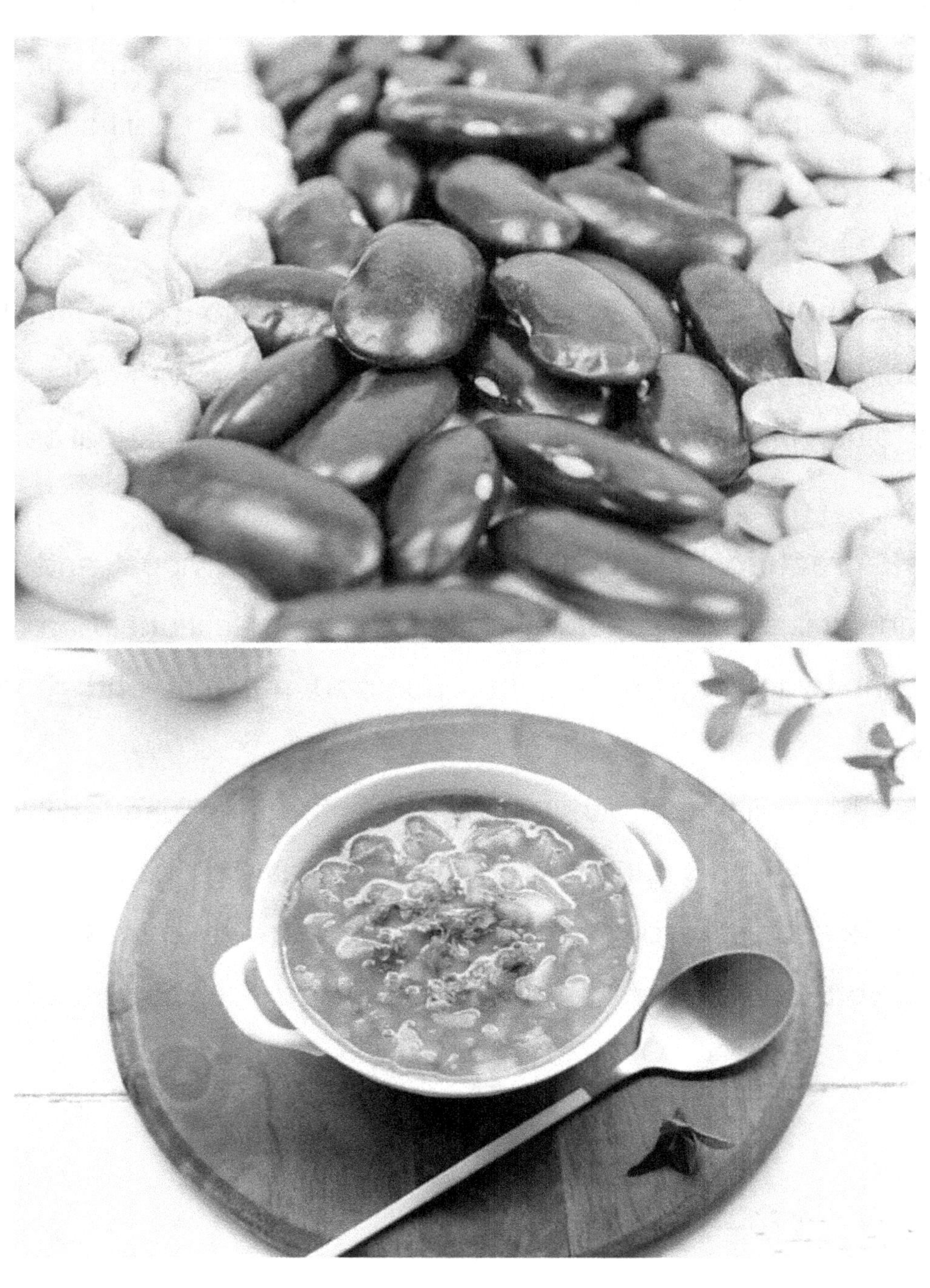

Chapter 3: Boosting Fertility Through Superfoods and Herbs

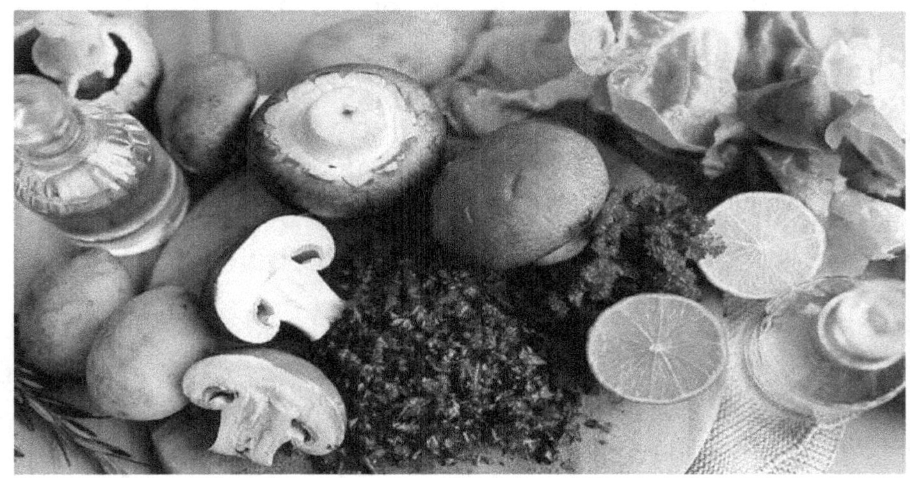

Fertility boosters such as superfoods and herbs are becoming increasingly popular among couples attempting to conceive. While these methods do not ensure pregnancy, they can improve general reproductive health and raise the odds of conception.

Superfoods are nutrient-dense foods that give a variety of health advantages, and some have been shown to improve fertility. Here are some superfoods that may aid in fertility:

Maca Root: This Peruvian root vegetable has long been used to boost fertility. Maca is high in vitamins, minerals, and amino acids, which help to balance hormones and boost the reproductive system.

Berries: Blueberries, raspberries, and strawberries are high in antioxidants, which neutralize free radicals and protect sperm and eggs. They also have folate, which promotes healthy cell division.

Leafy Greens: Spinach, kale, and other leafy greens are high in folate, iron, and calcium, all of which are essential for reproductive health. They are also abundant in antioxidants and fiber.

Whole Grains: Whole grains, such as quinoa, oats, and brown rice, are high in B vitamins, which are required for hormone production. They also give a consistent supply of energy and aid in blood sugar regulation.

Fatty Fish: Salmon, sardines, and mackerel are high in omega-3 fatty acids. These good fats aid in hormone regulation, inflammation reduction, and the formation of fertile cervical mucus.

Certain herbs, in addition to superfoods, have been used for generations to promote fertility. Here are a few herbs that are said to be beneficial to fertility:

Vitex: Vitex, also known as Chasteberry, has traditionally been used to regulate menstrual cycles and improve hormonal balance. It may aid in the treatment of illnesses including polycystic ovary syndrome (PCOS) and infertility caused by hormonal abnormalities.

Dong Quai: This Chinese herb has been used to regulate menstrual cycles and improve blood circulation to the reproductive organs. It is believed to strengthen the uterus and facilitate implantation.

Tribulus Terrestris: Commonly used in traditional Ayurvedic and Chinese medicine, Tribulus Terrestris may help enhance male fertility by increasing sperm count, motility, and quality.

Red Raspberry Leaf: This herb has been used for centuries to tone the reproductive system. It is believed to strengthen the uterus, regulate menstrual cycles, and improve fertility.

Before beginning any herbal regimen, it is critical to check with a healthcare expert or a qualified herbalist, especially if you have pre-existing health concerns or are taking medication. They can provide tailored advice based on your unique requirements and ensure that these herbs do not conflict with any existing therapies or diseases.

Remember that increasing fertility is a multifaceted task that includes living a healthy lifestyle, controlling stress, and seeking competent medical advice. Superfoods and herbs can help in this process, but it is critical to approach fertility with patience and knowledge.

A Guide to Fertility-Boosting Superfoods

Are you and your partner ready to take the plunge into parenthood? A healthy diet and prudent lifestyle choices can frequently help to increase fertility naturally. This article will look at a variety of superfoods that have been scientifically proven to improve fertility. These nutrient-dense powerhouses can supply critical vitamins, minerals, and antioxidants for reproductive health.

So join us as we explore the world of fertility-boosting superfoods and get one step closer to realizing your dream of starting a family.

Avocado: Avocados are high in heart-healthy monounsaturated fats and an excellent source of vitamin E. This vitamin has been linked to improved sperm quality and embryo implantation. Avocados are also high in folate, an important ingredient for a healthy pregnancy.

Berries: Strawberries, blueberries, and raspberries are antioxidant powerhouses that boost male and female fertility. Berries, which are high in Vitamin C and antioxidants, protect the eggs and sperm from oxidative damage, promoting healthy fertilization and conception.

Spinach: This leafy green is high in iron and folate, all of which are necessary for reproductive health. Iron aids in ovulation, whereas folate aids in the prevention of birth deformities and promotes a healthy sperm count. Including spinach in your diet can help you have a healthy pregnancy.

Salmon: High in omega-3 fatty acids, salmon maintains hormonal balance and increases fertility in both men and women. These healthy fats aid in menstruation regulation and enhance blood flow to the reproductive organs. These healthy fats aid in menstruation regulation and enhance blood flow to the reproductive organs. Salmon also includes vitamin D, which affects hormone production.

Pumpkin Seeds: These small but powerful seeds are high in critical nutrients like zinc and selenium. Zinc has been shown to boost sperm quality and induce ovulation, whereas selenium aids embryo growth and hormonal balance. For an added fertility boost, sprinkle pumpkin seeds on salads or blend them into smoothies.

Greek yogurt is high in protein and calcium, making it an excellent fertility food. Protein is essential for adequate hormone production, and calcium fosters a healthy uterine environment. Incorporating this superfood into your diet can benefit both couples.

Quinoa: Quinoa is a complete protein that contains all of the important amino acids required for reproductive health. It helps to keep blood sugar levels stable and menstrual periods regular, increasing the chances of pregnancy.

Walnuts: Walnuts, known as fertility boosters, are abundant in omega-3 fatty acids and antioxidants, which promote sperm quality and motility. Furthermore, walnuts are high in arginine, an amino acid that has been shown to improve blood flow to the reproductive organs.

When it comes to fertility, nutrition is extremely important. You can improve your chances of naturally conceiving by including these fertility-boosting superfoods in your diet. However, it is critical to remember that your dietary choices should be accompanied by a healthy and balanced lifestyle that includes frequent exercise and stress management. Always seek tailored guidance from a healthcare professional, and may your parenting journey be filled with joy and happiness.

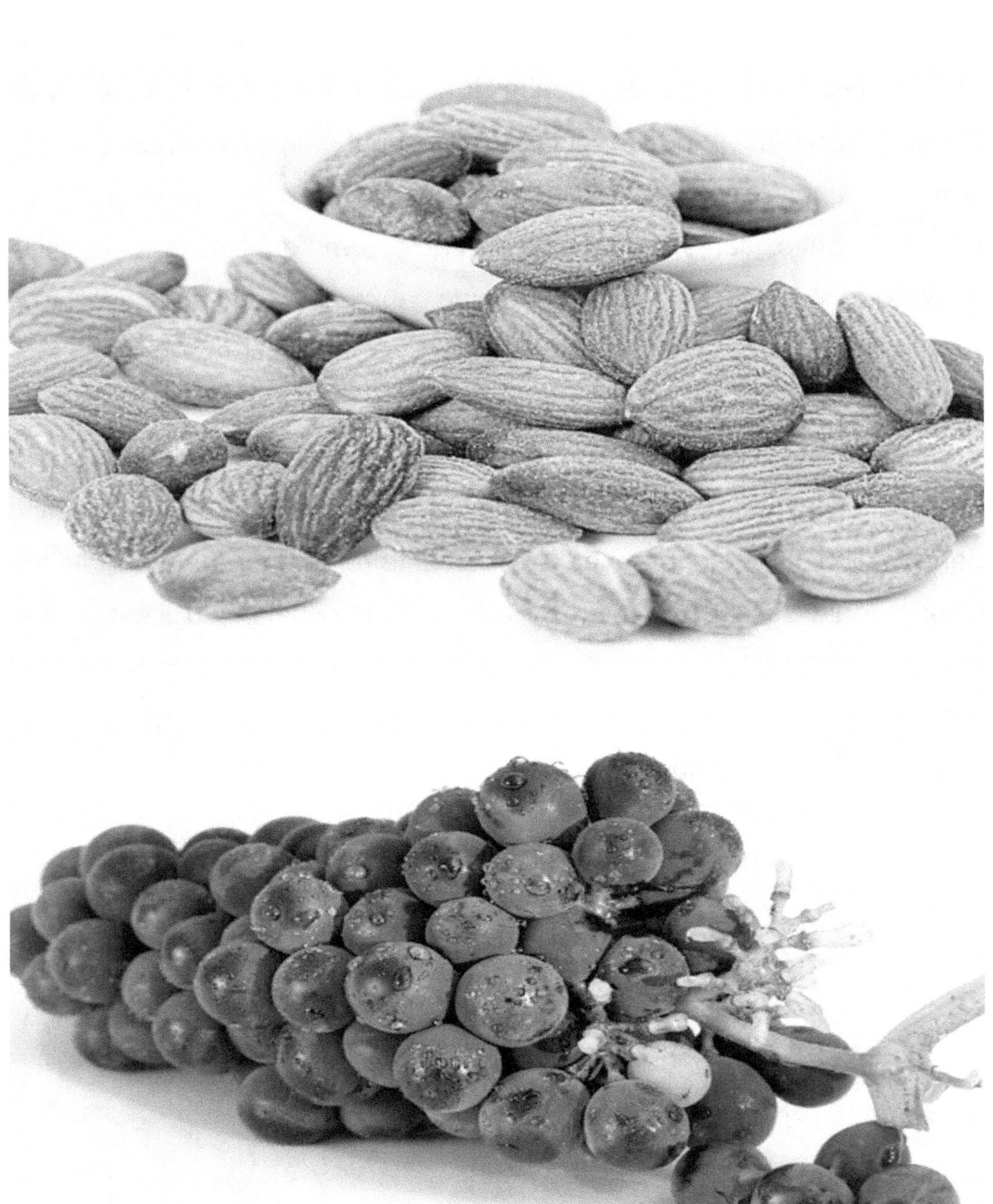

Plant-Based Proteins for Optimal Reproductive Health

Plant-based proteins have the potential to play an important role in promoting healthy reproductive health. Protein is a food that the body needs to generate hormones, grow and repair tissues, and sustain general biological processes. While animal-based proteins are frequently lauded for their nutritional content, plant-based proteins provide distinct advantages that can be beneficial to reproductive health.

The high fiber content of plant-based proteins is one of their main advantages. Fiber aids in digestion and the maintenance of good gut bacteria, which is essential for nutrition absorption and hormone balance. Furthermore, plant-based proteins are low in saturated fats, which can help with hormonal balance and overall cardiovascular health.

Certain plant-based proteins contain nutrients that are extremely important to reproductive health. Isoflavones, which are natural chemicals that act as phytoestrogens, are found in soy-based products such as tofu and tempeh. Phytoestrogens are known to imitate estrogen in the body and can help with a variety of reproductive health issues, including menopause symptoms and hormonal imbalances.

Legumes and beans are also high in plant-based proteins and critical elements like zinc and iron. These minerals are essential for reproductive health because they aid in the manufacture and transfer of reproductive hormones, normal cell division, and fetal development during pregnancy.

In addition, integrating a diversity of plant-based proteins into one's diet assures a variety of amino acids, which are the building blocks of protein.

Consuming a range of amino acids helps the body produce required proteins for reproductive health, such as enzymes that assist in digesting hormones and promote fertility.

While plant-based proteins have several benefits for reproductive health, it is critical to make informed dietary decisions and guarantee enough intake. Consultation with a healthcare expert or a qualified dietitian can assist in developing a well-balanced plant-based diet that meets protein requirements while also supporting optimal reproductive health.

Harnessing the Power of Adaptogens for Fertility Support

Adaptogens have grown in popularity as natural treatments for a variety of health issues, and harnessing their potency for reproductive assistance is an intriguing and promising topic. Fertility concerns can be emotionally draining for both people and couples, but adaptogens provide a comprehensive approach to improving reproductive health.

Adaptogens are a class of herbs and plants that have been utilized in traditional medicine for centuries. They have distinct features that assist the body in responding to stress, adapting to changes, and restoring balance. These herbs operate by balancing hormones, lowering inflammation, boosting the immune system, and improving overall health.

One of the most important ways adaptogens aid fertility is by lowering the impact of stress on the body. Stress can disturb the reproductive system by interfering with hormone homeostasis. Using adaptogens can assist in moderating the stress response, lower cortisol levels, and promote a more fertile environment.

Among the adaptogens renowned for their fertility-promoting qualities are:

- **Ashwagandha:** In Ayurvedic medicine, this plant is revered for its ability to decrease stress, balance hormones, and support reproductive function in both men and women.
- **Maca:** Maca root is high in antioxidants and important nutrients, which can help with hormonal balance, libido, and reproductive health.
- **Rhodiola Rosea:** This adaptogen is known for increasing energy and decreasing exhaustion, as well as promoting emotional well-being and maintaining hormonal balance.
- **Shatavari:** Ayurvedic medicine has traditionally employed Shatavari to control the menstrual cycle, promote female reproductive health, and boost fertility.
- **Eleuthero (Siberian Ginseng):** Eleuthero is an immune-stimulating adaptogen that promotes fertility by improving general health and well-being.

While adaptogens can help with fertility, it's vital to note that they should only be used in conjunction with a healthy lifestyle and under the supervision of a healthcare practitioner. Each individual's goals and circumstances are unique, and a skilled practitioner can assist in developing a customized approach to maximizing the benefits of adaptogens for conception support.

Finally, utilizing the potential of adaptogens for conception support can be an excellent addition to any reproductive health journey. They are a vital tool in optimizing fertility because of their capacity to relieve stress, balance hormones, and enhance overall well-being. However, to achieve the best results, they must be used in an informed and personalized manner.

Natural Herbs and Supplements to Enhance Fertility

Fertility is a major concern for many individuals and couples who are attempting to conceive. While there are numerous medical procedures and therapies available, some people prefer to use natural herbs and supplements to improve fertility. Although these herbs and supplements are generally thought to be safe, it is always recommended to talk with a healthcare expert before using them, especially if you have any underlying health concerns or are taking other medications.

The Maca Root

Maca root, often known as Peruvian ginseng, is a popular herb used to promote fertility. For millennia, it has been used to improve reproductive health and stimulate libido. Maca root is high in vitamins, minerals, and antioxidants, which can aid in hormone balance and overall reproductive health. It comes in powder form and can be used in smoothies or taken as a supplement.

Vitex

Vitex, often known as chaste tree berry, is a herb that is commonly used to balance hormones and promote conception. It works by increasing the production of luteinizing hormone (LH) and suppressing the release of follicle-stimulating hormone (FSH), which helps to regulate the menstrual cycle. Vitex is commonly taken in the form of capsules or tinctures.

Tribulus Terrestris 3.

Tribulus Terrestris is a herb that has been shown to increase fertility in both men and women. Traditional medicine has used it to boost libido, enhance sperm count in men, and balance hormone levels. Tribulus terrestris is often taken as a supplement in the form of a pill or powder.

Leaf of Red Raspberry

Red raspberry leaf is a well-known plant for its ability to strengthen the uterus and increase fertility. It is high in vitamins, minerals, and antioxidants, all of which are beneficial to reproductive health. Red raspberry leaf tea is a popular way to ingest this herb, and it is generally regarded as safe for the majority of individuals.

Coenzyme Q10 (CoQ10) is a type of antioxidant.

Coenzyme Q10 is a potent antioxidant that aids in the creation of energy within cells. According to research, it may help increase egg and sperm quality, particularly in people undergoing reproductive procedures such as in vitro fertilization (IVF). CoQ10 is available as a supplement in the form of capsules or tablets.

DHEA

The adrenal glands produce the hormone dehydroepiandrosterone (DHEA). DHEA supplementation has been found to promote fertility and increase the odds of a successful pregnancy, particularly in women with a low ovarian reserve. DHEA is often taken in the form of a capsule or tablet.

While natural herbs and supplements can help with fertility, they should not be used as the primary treatment for infertility. Maintaining a healthy diet, engaging in regular exercise, managing stress levels, and seeking medical counsel for any underlying health concerns that may be influencing fertility are all crucial. Consultation with a reproductive medicine specialist is essential for designing a tailored approach based on your specific needs and circumstances.

Superfood Recipes to Nourish Your Fertility

Berry Blast Smoothie:

1 cup mixed berries (blueberries, strawberries, and raspberries), 1 ripe banana, 1 cup spinach, 1 cup almond milk, and 1 tablespoon chia seeds.

Directions: Blend all ingredients until smooth. This smoothie is high in antioxidants, folate, and vitamins that are beneficial to reproductive health.

Quinoa Salad:

1 cup cooked quinoa, 1 cup mixed veggies (broccoli, bell peppers, and carrots), 1/4 cup chopped walnuts, 1/4 cup dried cranberries, 2 tablespoons extra-virgin olive oil, 1 tablespoon lemon juice, salt and pepper to taste.

Direction: Toss all of the ingredients together in a mixing basin. Quinoa contains protein, iron, and fiber, all of which are necessary for reproductive health.

Avocado Toast:

2 slices of whole-grain bread, 1 ripe avocado, 1 teaspoon of lemon juice, salt, and pepper to taste.

Directions: Toast the slices of bread till golden brown. Combine the avocado, lemon juice, salt, and pepper in a mixing bowl. On the toast, spread the avocado mixture. Avocados are high in healthy fats and vitamin E, both of which boost fertility.

Salmon with Roasted Vegetables:

2 salmon fillets, 1 tablespoon olive oil, 2 cups mixed veggies (such as sweet potatoes, zucchini, and asparagus), salt and pepper to taste. **Directions:** Preheat the oven to 400 degrees Fahrenheit (200 degrees Celsius). Toss the vegetables in a bowl with olive oil, salt, and pepper. For 20-25 minutes, roast the vegetables. Season the salmon with salt and pepper before baking it for 12-15 minutes, or until it is cooked through.

Salmon contains omega-3 fatty acids, which can help with fertility.

Remember that, while these superfoods can help with fertility, it's always important to maintain a healthy lifestyle and get tailored counsel from a healthcare practitioner. On your way to a happy and healthy pregnancy, try these delectable and nourishing meals.

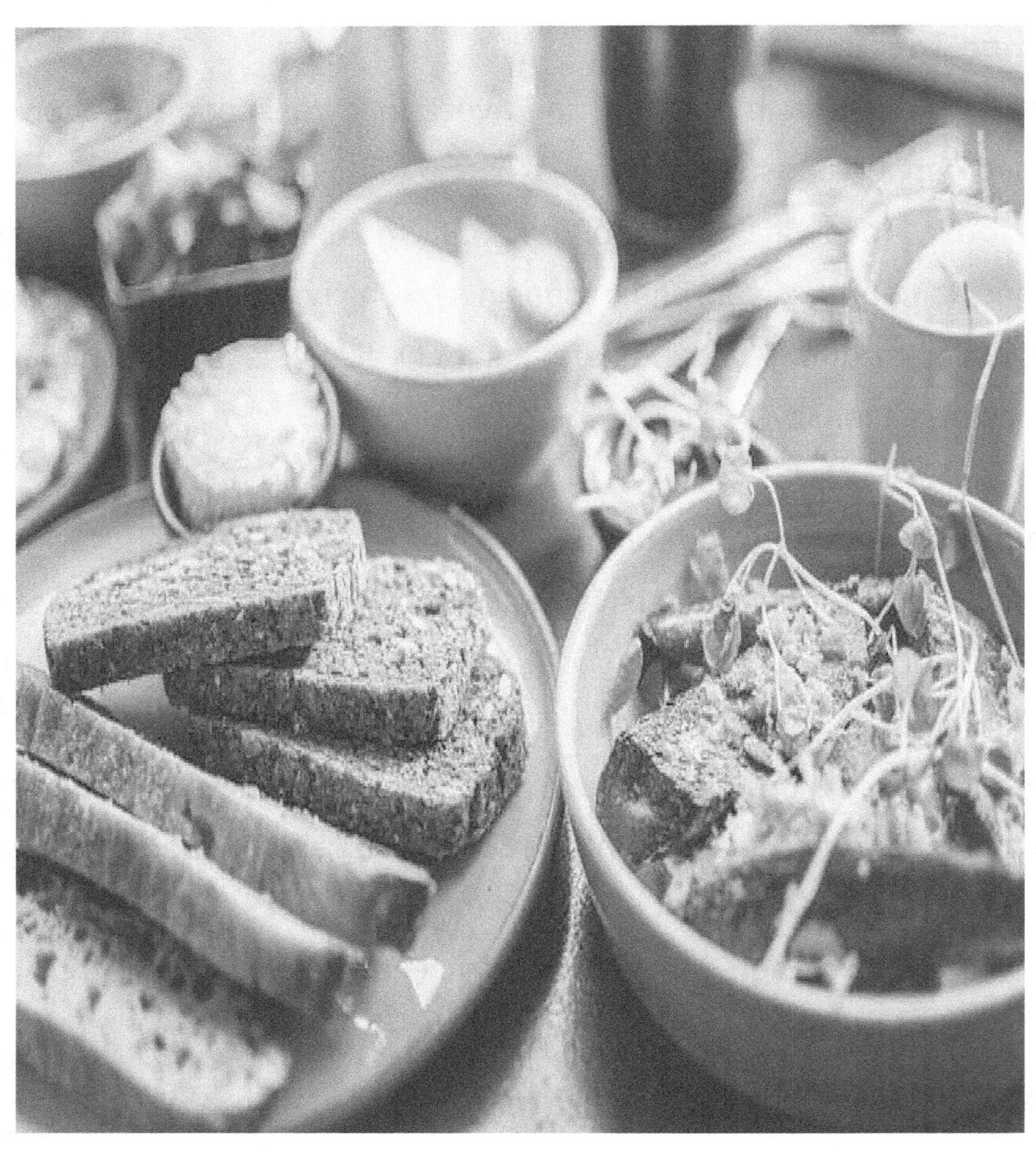

Chapter 4: Meal Planning and Recipes for Enhanced Fertility

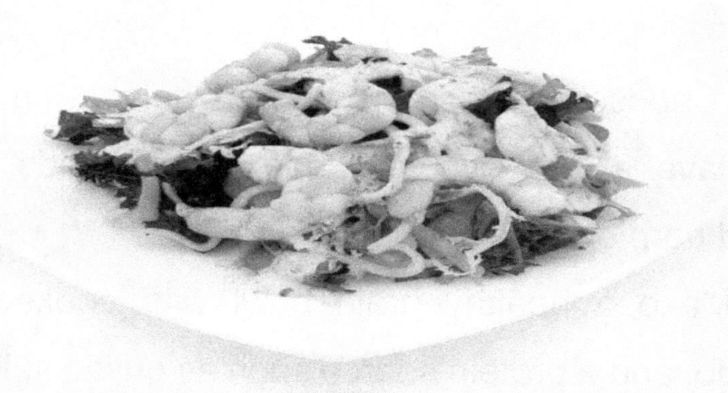

Meal planning and recipes can be quite beneficial in boosting increased fertility. A well-balanced diet rich in nutrients can assist maintain reproductive health and boost the chances of conception. Furthermore, the appropriate balance of vitamins, minerals, and antioxidants can improve both male and female fertility. Here are some healthful foods and recipe ideas to consider when meal planning for increased fertility.

Leafy Greens: Include lots of leafy greens in your meals, such as spinach, kale, and Swiss chard. These vegetables are high in folate, a B vitamin that promotes healthy cell division and can help with embryonic development.
Recipe idea: Make a delectable spinach salad with fresh berries, almonds, and a balsamic vinaigrette. Kale can also be sautéed with garlic and served as a side dish.

Colored Fruits and Veggies: Include a range of colored fruits and veggies in your fertility diet. Berries, tomatoes, carrots, and bell peppers are high in antioxidants, which can help fight oxidative stress.

Recipe idea: Make a nutritious mixed fruit salad or a colorful stir-fry with a variety of veggies and lean protein like chicken or tofu.

Whole Grains: Choose whole grains such as quinoa, brown rice, and oats. These grains have a low glycemic index, which aids with blood sugar stabilization and hormonal balance.

Recipe idea: Make a healthy grain bowl with cooked quinoa, roasted veggies, avocado, and a protein source such as grilled salmon or chickpeas.

Lean Proteins: Include lean protein sources including poultry, fish, eggs, and lentils in your diet. Protein is essential for fertility since it contains the amino acids required for hormone production and overall reproductive health.

Recipe idea: Prepare a healthful supper by grilling chicken breasts and serving them with steamed vegetables and quinoa on the side.

Healthy Fats: Include healthy fats in your diet, such as avocados, nuts, seeds, and olive oil. These lipids are necessary for the generation and function of hormones.

Recipe idea: Make a tasty avocado and mixed nut salad or sprinkle olive oil over roasted vegetables for extra flavor.

Remember that, while meal planning is vital for fertility, it is also important to have an overall healthy lifestyle. This involves regular physical activity, stress management, and avoiding excessive caffeine and alcohol consumption. To get individualized counsel and guidance targeted to your specific needs, it's always a good idea to talk with a healthcare expert or a registered dietitian who specializes in fertility nutrition.

The Basics of Smart Meal Planning for Fertility

Smart fertility meal planning focuses on improving nutrition to increase fertility in both men and women. It entails choosing and adding fertility-friendly items to your diet while also ensuring that your general nutritional needs are met. Here are some fundamentals to get you started:

- **Balanced and Nutrient-Rich Meals:** It is critical to consume a well-balanced and nutrient-rich diet to boost fertility. Include fruits, vegetables, whole grains, lean proteins, and healthy fats in your diet. Choose foods rich in vitamins, minerals, and antioxidants, such as leafy greens, berries, nuts, seeds, and legumes.

- **Emphasize Healthy Fats:** Healthy fats are essential for hormone production and should be included in your diet. Include avocados, olive oil, coconut oil, nuts, seeds, and fatty seafood such as salmon. These fats also help in the absorption of fat-soluble vitamins, such as vitamin D, which is necessary for fertility.

- **Adequate Protein Intake:** Protein is required for the creation of reproductive hormones as well as the generation of healthy eggs and sperm. Include lean protein sources in your meals, such as fowl, fish, beans, lentils, and tofu. However, heavy consumption of red and processed meats has been linked to reduced fertility.

- **Increase Antioxidant Intake:** Antioxidants protect the reproductive organs from oxidative stress and free radical damage. Consume antioxidant-rich foods such as berries, citrus fruits, dark leafy greens, tomatoes, nuts, and seeds. Include bright vegetables and fruits that are high in vitamins, minerals, and bioactive substances.

- **Fiber-Rich Foods:** A fiber-rich diet aids in blood sugar regulation and general hormonal balance. Increase your fiber intake by eating whole grains, legumes, fruits, vegetables, and seeds. Fiber-rich foods also aid in the maintenance of a healthy weight, which is essential for fertility.

- **Limit Processed Foods and Added Sugars:** Processed foods frequently contain harmful fats, added sugars, and artificial additives that might interfere with hormonal balance. Reduce your intake of processed foods and sugary snacks, as these may impair fertility. Instead, choose complete, unprocessed foods that are high in nutrients.

- **Hydration:** Maintaining appropriate hydration is critical for general health and fertility. Throughout the day, drink lots of water. Herbal teas, infused water, and fresh fruit juices with no additional sugars can also be included if desired.

Remember that, while eating is crucial for fertility, it is equally necessary to live a healthy lifestyle, exercise regularly, get adequate sleep, and reduce stress. Consultation with a healthcare professional, such as a dietitian or fertility specialist, can provide tailored advice and assistance.

Breakfast Recipes for Hormonal Balance

Breakfast is the most important meal of the day, and it is even more vital when it comes to hormonal balance. Hormones are essential in the regulation of several body activities, including metabolism, mood, and energy levels. Here are some delicious and nutritious breakfast recipes that help with hormone balance:

1. Superfood Smoothie Bowl: Combine a handful of spinach, a frozen banana, a scoop of antioxidant-rich berries (such as blueberries or raspberries), a dollop of almond butter, a tablespoon of chia seeds, and a cup of almond milk in a blender. Pour the smoothie into a bowl and top with sliced fruits, nuts, and seeds for extra crunch. The combination of vibrant fruits, healthy fats, and fiber-rich ingredients will keep your hormones happy and your taste buds satisfied.

2. Avocado and Egg Toast: Start by toasting a slice of whole-grain bread and mashing half an avocado onto it. Sprinkle some red pepper flakes, sea salt, and black pepper for extra flavor. In a separate pan, cook an egg until it is sunny-side up or in whichever way you prefer. Place the egg on top of the avocado toast and, if desired, add some fresh herbs like cilantro or parsley. Avocado is rich in healthy fats, while eggs are a great source of proteins and vitamin D, both essential for hormone balance.

3. Quinoa Breakfast Bowl: Cook the quinoa according to package directions. In a separate pan, sauté some chopped vegetables such as bell peppers, spinach, and mushrooms. Once tender, combine the cooked quinoa with the sautéed vegetables. Add a sprinkle of turmeric, cumin, and paprika for extra flavor. To make it more satisfying, top it with crumbled feta cheese or avocado slices. This nutrient-dense breakfast is high in protein, fiber, and a range of vitamins and minerals, all of which can help with hormonal balance.

4. Greek Yogurt Parfait: Layer plain Greek yogurt with an array of fruits such as berries, sliced bananas, and mangoes in a bowl or glass. Sprinkle with granola and drizzle with honey to serve. Greek yogurt is high in protein, which can assist in regulating blood sugar levels and hormones. Fruit's inherent sweetness complements the creamy yogurt, making it an ideal breakfast option for hormonal balance.

5. Veggie Omelette: Whisk together two eggs and a splash of milk in a mixing bowl. Heat a teaspoon of olive oil in a nonstick skillet over medium heat. Pour in the egg mixture and heat until the borders are firm but the middle is still somewhat runny. To one side of the omelet, add a handful of chopped veggies such as spinach, tomatoes, and bell peppers. Fold the other side over the veggies after the eggs are fully cooked. For a complete meal, serve it with whole-grain toast. This protein-rich omelet, combined with the fiber from the vegetables and complex carbohydrates from the toast, provides for a filling and hormonally balanced breakfast.

Remember that the key to maintaining hormonal balance is to eat a varied and balanced diet full of healthful ingredients high in important nutrients. So try these breakfast recipes for a wonderful start to your day while also nourishing your hormonal health.

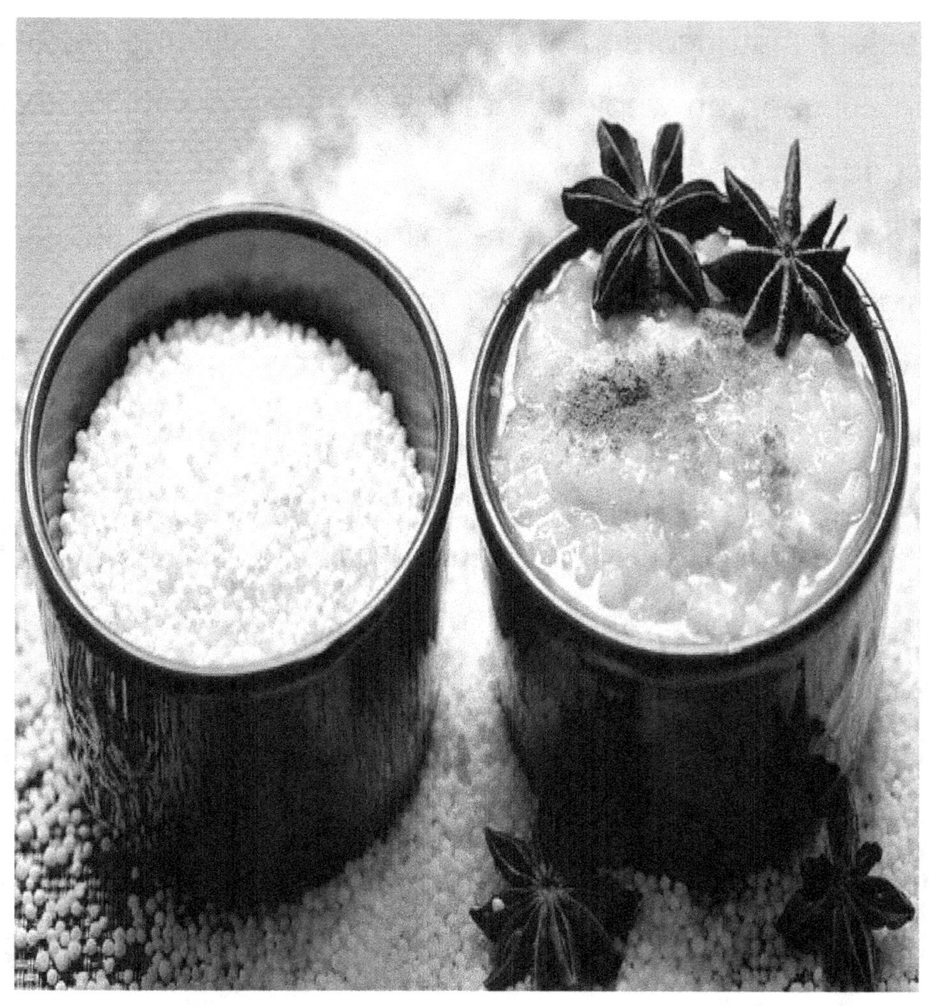

Nourishing Lunches and Snacks to Boost Fertility

Maintaining a balanced and nutrient-rich diet can play an important role in increasing fertility. Taking care of your body and feeding it the correct foods can improve your reproductive health. Incorporating nutritious foods and snacks into your diet can be both tasty and beneficial to your reproductive quest. Here are some suggestions to get you started:

1. Avocado Toast with Spinach and Eggs: Begin your day with a nutrient-dense breakfast that incorporates healthy fats, leafy greens, and protein. Spread ripe avocado on whole wheat toast, then top with sautéed spinach and a poached egg for added protein.

2. Berry Smoothie Bowl: Berries are not only vibrant and pleasant, but they are also high in antioxidants, which can help with general reproductive health. Blend some mixed berries, Greek yogurt, spinach, and almond milk. Pour the smoothie into a bowl and top with your preferred nuts, seeds, and oats for a filling and fertility-friendly snack.

3. Quinoa Salad with Roasted Vegetables: Quinoa is a high-protein, fiber-rich grain that is also abundant in vital minerals. Roast bright veggies like bell peppers, zucchini, and sweet potatoes. Toss them with cooked quinoa and a lemon vinaigrette dressing for a robust salad that is not only tasty but also beneficial to fertility.

4. Nut Butter Energy Balls: Make your energy balls with your favorite nut butter, oats, chia seeds, and a drizzle of honey. These small bites include a good balance of healthy fats, fiber, and protein. Refrigerate them for a quick and healthful snack in between meals.

Remember that healthy eating habits go hand in hand with healthy living practices. Regular exercise, stress management strategies, and adequate rest all contribute to general well-being and improve fertility. So, in addition to integrating these nourishing lunches and snacks into your diet, keep a holistic approach in mind to enhance your reproductive journey.

Wholesome Dinners for Optimal Reproductive Health

Eating nutritious dinners is essential for good reproductive health. Here are some ideas for eating a healthy, balanced diet that will help your reproductive system:

- **Salmon:** High in omega-3 fatty acids, salmon aids in hormone regulation and conception. For a filling dinner, serve baked or grilled salmon fillets with steamed veggies.

- **Leafy greens:** Include nutrient-dense greens such as spinach, kale, and Swiss chard in your diet. These greens are high in folate, iron, and calcium, all of which are necessary for reproductive health. Make a nutritious salad with them or stir-fry them with other colorful vegetables.

- **Quinoa:** This grain-like seed is high in plant protein and vital amino acids. For a well-rounded dinner, prepare a nutritious quinoa bowl with roasted veggies and a protein of your choosing.

- **Berries:** High in antioxidants, berries such as blueberries, strawberries, and raspberries can help protect eggs and sperm from free radical damage. Serve them as a refreshing dessert or toss them into a green salad for a taste boost.

- **Lean proteins:** Choose lean protein sources such as chicken breast, tofu, or lentils. Protein is essential for the formation of healthy reproductive tissues.

- **Whole grains:** Whole grains are high in fiber and important nutrients, such as brown rice, whole wheat bread, and oats. They control insulin levels, which are important for reproductive health. For dinner, make a nice grain-based salad or a filling dish of warm oatmeal with strawberries.

- **Nuts and seeds:** Almonds, walnuts, chia seeds, and flaxseeds are high in omega-3 fatty acids and good fats. For a healthy dose of deliciousness, sprinkle them over a salad or combine them into a homemade trail mix.

Remember to seek tailored advice on reproductive health and any unique dietary requirements from a healthcare practitioner or certified dietitian.

Indulgent yet Fertility-Friendly Dessert Ideas

Indulging in desserts while adhering to a fertility-friendly diet may be a pleasant and delectable challenge. Fortunately, several scrumptious dessert options will please your sweet craving while also helping you achieve your fertility goals. Consider the following inventive and delectable alternatives:

- **Superfood Smoothie Bowl:** A smoothie bowl is a nutritious and visually beautiful dessert concept that is also good for fertility. Begin by combining a mixture of fertility-friendly fruits such as berries, bananas, and mangoes. Then add superfoods like chia seeds, flaxseeds, almonds, and coconut flakes on top.

- **Dark Chocolate Covered Berries:** Chocolate and berries are a delicious combo, and dark chocolate in particular can help with fertility. Melt dark chocolate and dip strawberries, raspberries, or blueberries in it to indulge. Refrigerate until the chocolate solidifies, then serve this sweet and antioxidant-rich treat.

- **Greek Yogurt Parfait:** A delightful and nutrient-dense dessert that can be made by layering Greek yogurt, granola, and fertility-friendly fruits like pomegranate seeds, bananas, or kiwis. Greek yogurt is high in protein and calcium, both of which are beneficial to reproductive health.

- **Avocado Chocolate Mousse:** Avocado is a versatile and nutrient-dense fruit that works well as a foundation for creamy sweets. Combine ripe avocados, dark chocolate powder, a natural sweetener like honey or maple syrup, and a splash of vanilla essence in a mixing bowl. This rich and velvety chocolate mousse is not only decadent but also high in heart-healthy fats and antioxidants.

- **Cinnamon-Spiced Baked Apples:** Baked apples are a simple yet delicious dessert, especially when seasoned with fertility-friendly spices like cinnamon. Bake until the apples are tender after being cored and stuffed with oats, almonds, and cinnamon. The natural sweetness of the apples, mixed with the comforting scents of cinnamon, combine to make a warm and pleasant delicacy.

Even with fertility-friendly treats, moderation is crucial. These decadent ideas can be enjoyed as part of a well-balanced diet that promotes fertility.

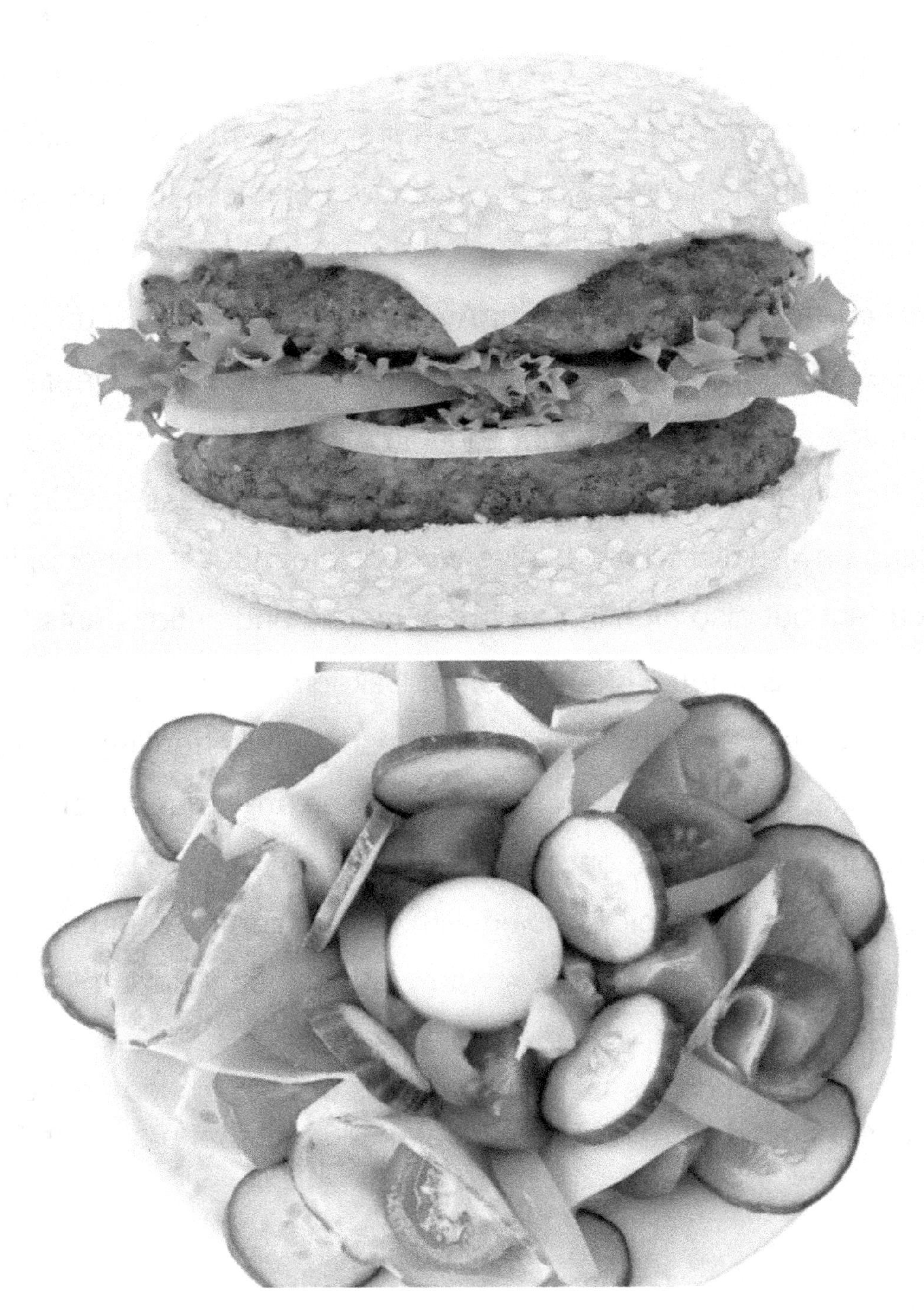

Chapter 5: Lifestyle Modifications for Increased Fertility

Lifestyle changes can significantly increase fertility and improve your chances of conceiving. You can improve your reproductive health and increase your chances of a successful pregnancy by making certain modifications to your daily routine and habits. Consider the following lifestyle changes for higher fertility:

Maintain a Healthy Weight: Both being underweight and being overweight can hurt fertility. Aim for a healthy BMI by eating a balanced diet, exercising regularly, and checking with a healthcare expert as needed.

Eat a Nutritious Diet: A well-balanced, nutrient-rich diet helps improve fertility. Consume plenty of whole grains, fruits and vegetables, lean proteins, and healthy fats. Incorporating fertility-boosting foods such as avocado, walnuts, leafy greens, and antioxidant-rich berries can also help.

Avoid Harmful Substances: Reduce or eliminate your usage of substances that can impair fertility. Tobacco, alcohol, and recreational drugs are examples of this. It has been demonstrated that smoking and heavy alcohol intake reduce fertility in both men and women.

Manage Stress: Stress can have a detrimental influence on fertility by disturbing hormone balance. Incorporating stress-reduction practices such as meditation, yoga, or any other activity that helps you relax will help you become more fertile.

Regular Exercise: Regular moderate-intensity exercise can help with reproductive health. Exercise promotes a healthy weight, increases blood supply to reproductive organs, and reduces stress. However, don't overdo it, as too much exercise can have a detrimental impact on fertility.

While there is no agreement on the specific amount of caffeine that impacts fertility, it is generally recommended to limit caffeine use to moderate levels. This includes limiting your intake of coffee, tea, energy drinks, and soda.

Get Adequate Sleep: Aim for 7-8 hours of quality sleep per night. Adequate rest aids in hormone regulation and enhances overall reproductive health.

Maintaining a regular and healthy sexual life can boost your chances of conceiving. Throughout your menstrual cycle, try to have intercourse every two to three days, especially during your fertile window.

Making lifestyle changes can improve fertility and enhance your chances of conception. Remember to seek specialized guidance from a healthcare practitioner, especially if you have any underlying medical concerns affecting fertility.

The Role of Exercise in Promoting Female Fertility

Exercise can help increase female fertility by improving overall reproductive health and increasing the odds of conception. Physical activity regularly has been shown to improve hormonal balance, menstrual regularity, and blood circulation, all of which are important for reproductive health.

1. Hormone Balance: Exercise aids in the maintenance of a healthy weight, which is essential for hormonal balance. Obesity or significant weight gain can cause hormonal imbalances, resulting in irregular menstrual periods and decreased fertility. Regular exercise, particularly cardiovascular sports such as running, swimming, or cycling, can aid in the regulation of hormones such as estrogen and progesterone, which are required for ovulation and the maintenance of a healthy reproductive system.

2. Increased Blood Circulation: Exercise increases blood flow to reproductive organs, which improves their functionality. Improved blood circulation aids in the delivery of essential nutrients and oxygen to the ovaries, enabling healthy egg formation. Furthermore, exercise causes the release of endorphins, or "feel-good" hormones, which can help reduce stress and promote relaxation; stress has been shown to hurt fertility.

3. Stress Management: Stress is a well-known element that might interfere with conception. Regular exercise can help produce endorphins, enhance mood, and reduce anxiety, making it an effective stress reliever. Women can proactively manage stress and enhance their general well-being by including exercise in their regimen, ultimately laying the groundwork for healthy fertility.

4. Improving Body Composition: Maintaining a healthy body composition through exercise can positively influence fertility. Excessive body fat can disrupt the delicate balance of hormones responsible for ovulation, while low body fat percentage can lead to irregular or absent menstrual cycles. Regular physical activity, combined with a balanced diet, can help maintain healthy body weight and composition, creating an environment conducive to fertility. While physical activity is typically favorable for female fertility, excessive or severe physical activity might have the reverse impact. Extreme exercise regimens, such as severe endurance training or an excess of high-impact activities, can cause irregular menstrual cycles or even amenorrhea (lack of periods). It's critical to create a balance and listen to your body's needs, ensuring you work out within your boundaries.

Overall, including regular exercise in a woman's lifestyle can benefit her fertility by supporting hormonal balance, improving blood circulation, stress management, and keeping a healthy body composition. Pairing exercise with a balanced diet and other healthy lifestyle choices can greatly increase the chances of conception and contribute to overall reproductive health.

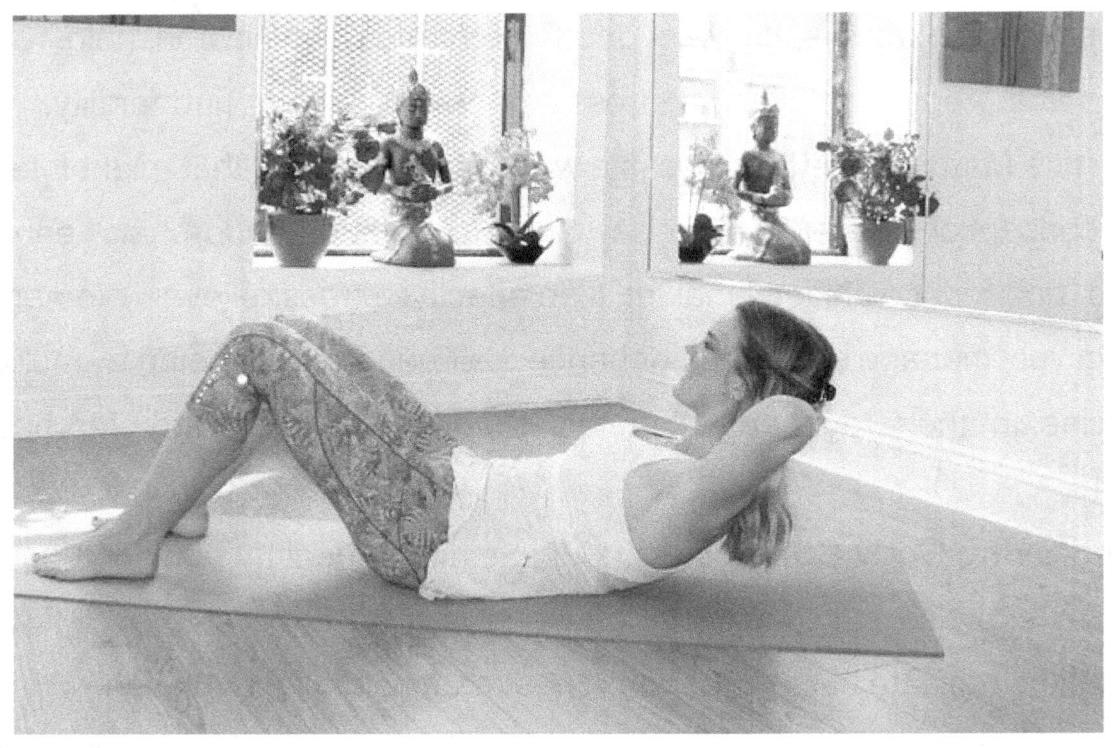

Stress Management Techniques for Optimal Reproductive Health

Stress management techniques play a crucial role in maintaining optimal reproductive health. High levels of stress can have negative effects on the hormonal balance and function of the reproductive system. To ensure that your reproductive health is well-maintained, here are some effective stress management techniques:

- **Exercise Regularly:** Engaging in physical activity has been proven to reduce stress levels and promote overall well-being. Regular exercise releases endorphins, which are known to boost mood and lower stress. Aim for at least 30 minutes of moderate-intensity exercise, such as jogging, swimming, or yoga, several times a week.

- **Practice Mindfulness and Meditation:** Mindfulness and meditation techniques are effective in calming the mind and reducing stress. Taking a few minutes each day to sit quietly and focus on your breath can help alleviate anxiety and promote relaxation. Apps like Headspace or Calm can guide you through meditation exercises if you are new to the practice.

- **Get Sufficient Sleep:** Prioritizing quality sleep is essential for managing stress and maintaining reproductive health. Lack of sleep can disrupt hormone production and increase stress levels. Aim for 7-8 hours of uninterrupted sleep each night and establish a regular sleep routine.

- **Seek Emotional Support:** Sharing your feelings and concerns with trusted individuals, such as a partner, friend, or therapist, can help relieve stress and restore emotional balance. A strong support system can provide encouragement, advice, and understanding during challenging times.

- **Engage in Relaxation Techniques:** Incorporate relaxation techniques like deep breathing exercises, progressive muscle relaxation, or aromatherapy into your daily routine. Experiment with different techniques to find what works best for you in reducing stress and promoting relaxation.

- **Prioritize Self-Care:** Make time for activities that bring you joy and help you de-stress. Engaging in hobbies, reading, listening to music, taking baths, or stepping into nature can all contribute to a sense of well-being. Taking care of yourself physically, emotionally, and mentally is vital for managing stress effectively.

- **Practice Time Management:** Feeling overwhelmed and stressed can happen when there is too much on your plate. Learn to manage your time effectively by prioritizing tasks, breaking them down into manageable chunks, and delegating when appropriate. Setting boundaries and learning to say "no" can also relieve pressure and prevent stress overload.

Remember, every individual's stress management needs are different, so it's important to find techniques that work best for you. By incorporating these stress management practices into your daily life, you can promote optimal reproductive health and overall well-being.

Sleep and its Impact on Fertility

Sleep is an essential part of our daily routine that affects many elements of our health, including fertility. Sleep involves a complex set of physiological and neurological actions that help repair our body and mind. Our reproductive system obtains the required support during this repair time, altering fertility.

Sleep has a significant impact on fertility by regulating hormone production. Sleep deprivation or irregular sleep patterns might upset the delicate hormonal balance required for reproductive health. Inadequate sleep, for example, can cause an increase in the hormone cortisol, which can interfere with the production of luteinizing hormone (LH) and follicle-stimulating hormone (FSH), both of which are required for egg development and ovulation in women and sperm generation in men.

Furthermore, sleep is essential for the general functioning of our reproductive system. Inadequate sleep can impair immunological function, rendering people more vulnerable to illnesses that might harm fertility. Chronic sleep deprivation is also linked to increased inflammation, which can damage the reproductive system. Furthermore, lack of sleep can have an impact on sperm quality by lowering sperm count, motility, and morphology. The circadian rhythm, our internal biological clock that regulates a variety of physical activities, including sleep, is intimately tied to fertility. Disruptions in this cycle, such as irregular sleep schedules or working night shifts, can upset the natural hormonal balance and harm reproductive health. Inconsistent sleep patterns, for example, have been linked to menstrual cycle irregularities and anovulation, making it difficult for women to conceive. Taking care of sleep difficulties and enhancing sleep quality can help improve reproductive outcomes. A regular sleep pattern can assist in controlling the circadian cycle and improve hormonal equilibrium. Creating a sleep-friendly environment, providing comfortable bedding, and keeping the room cold and dark can all help you get better sleep.

Aside from sleep, it is critical to consider and manage any underlying health issues or lifestyle variables that may contribute to sleep difficulties. Stress, obesity, sleep disorders such as sleep apnea, and certain drugs can all affect sleep quality and fertility.

Overall, prioritizing sleep and getting enough quality sleep is essential for preserving reproductive health and enhancing fertility results. Recognizing the link between sleep and fertility is critical, as is making conscious steps to improve sleep habits for people wishing to conceive.

I hope you find this book beneficial. Do you want a special vegetable garden directly in your home to help you receive enough nutrients, save money, and beautify your home?
I have a detailed step-by-step book named "Vegetable Gardening for Beginners" that provides vital knowledge and direction on how to establish and manage a successful vegetable garden.

CLICK HERE TO GET VEGETABLE GARDENING FOR BEGINNERS

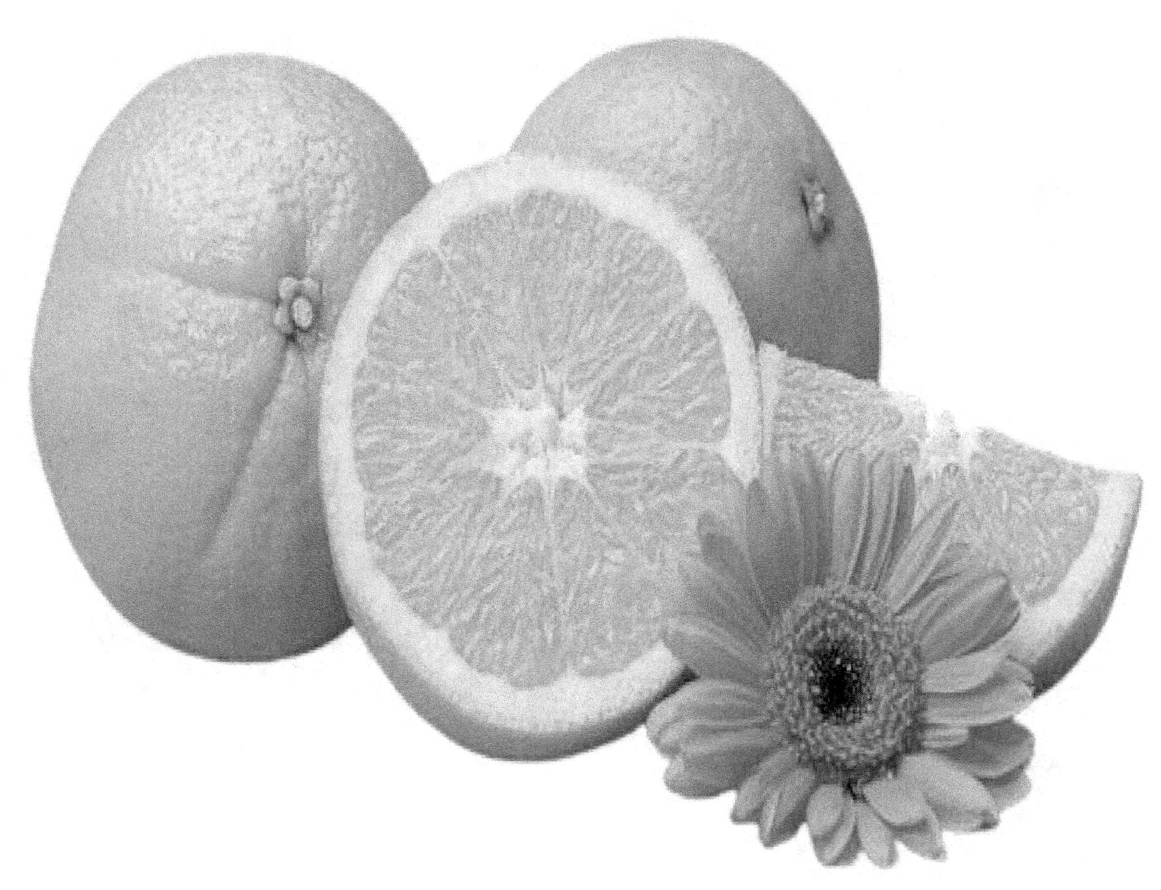

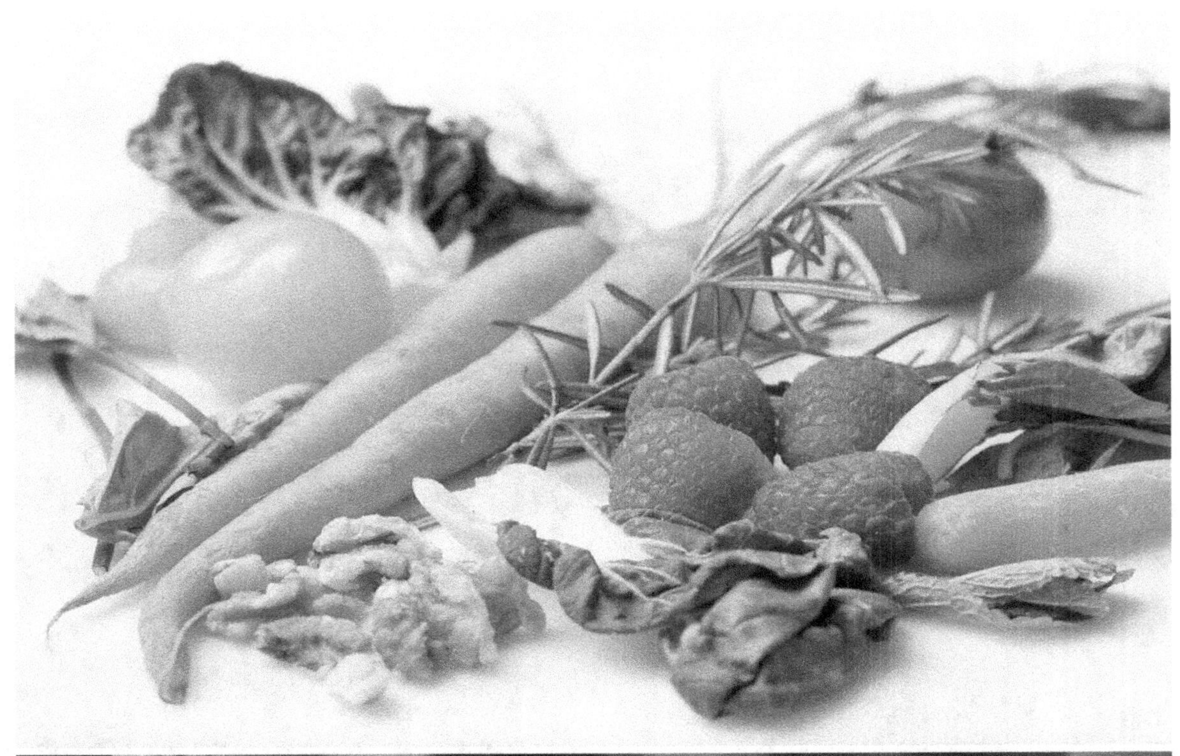

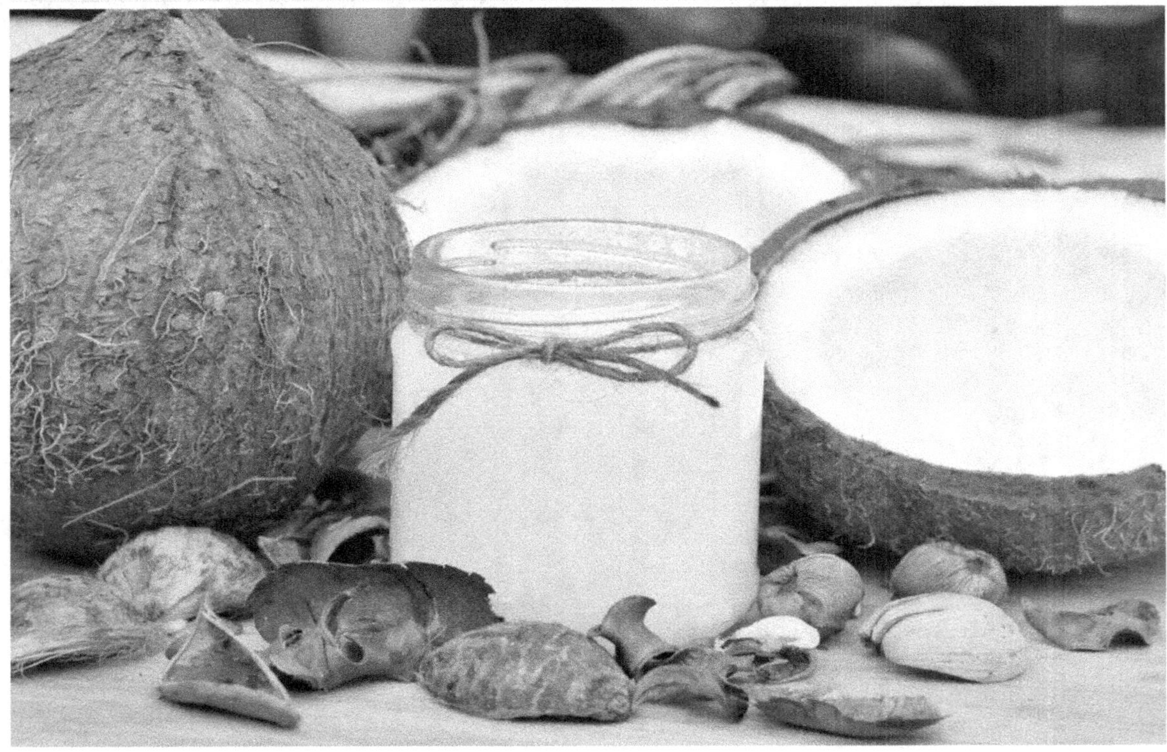

Mindfulness and Meditation Practices for Fertility Support

Mindfulness and meditation activities, which help individuals establish a state of calm, focused awareness and increase general emotional well-being, can be a valuable tool to assist fertility. This is especially useful for coping with stress, worry, and the emotional issues that are often connected with infertility struggles.

Bringing one's attention to the present moment, completely experiencing and accepting it without judgment, is what mindfulness entails. Individuals who practice mindfulness can learn to examine their thoughts, feelings, and body sensations in a more objective and non-reactive manner. This can help individuals escape the loop of negative or anxious thinking, allowing them to approach their reproductive journey with better clarity and equanimity. Conscious breathing is a method commonly employed in mindfulness meditation. This is concentrating on the breath and observing the feelings as air enters and exits the body. Individuals can develop a sense of grounding and relaxation by intentionally directing attention to the breath, lowering the physical and mental tension usually linked with fertility stress.

Body scan meditation is another popular type of mindfulness meditation. This entails paying attention to different sections of the body in a systematic manner and monitoring any physical sensations or tension without judgment. Individuals can build a deeper connection with their physical and mental states by tuning into the body's signals, helping them to better recognize and manage potential underlying imbalances influencing fertility.

In addition to these techniques, visualization and guided imagery exercises for reproductive support can be incorporated into mindfulness and meditation practices. Visualization is imagining favorable fertility outcomes, such as a healthy pregnancy or childbirth. Guided imagery exercises employ spoken instructions or recorded scripts to relax people so they may picture certain scenarios or imagery related to their fertility goals.

Some people may opt to engage in concurrent holistic practices to maximize the advantages of mindfulness and meditation in the setting of fertility. This could include incorporating relaxation techniques into their practice, such as gentle yoga or progressive muscular relaxation.

This may include integrating relaxation techniques, such as gentle yoga or progressive muscle relaxation, into their practice. Physical activity and exercise can be beneficial for overall health and stress reduction, which can indirectly support fertility.

It is important to note that while mindfulness and meditation practices can provide valuable support to individuals on their fertility journey, they should be seen as complementary to, rather than a substitute for, medical interventions. They can help individuals cope with the emotional toll of fertility struggles, but it is essential to consult with a healthcare provider for a comprehensive approach to fertility support.

In summary, mindfulness and meditation practices can be a valuable tools in supporting fertility by promoting emotional well-being, managing stress, and fostering a sense of balance and acceptance. By incorporating practices like conscious breathing, body scan meditation, visualization, and guided imagery, individuals can cultivate a greater sense of calm and resilience, enhancing their overall fertility experience.

Achieving Work-Life Balance to Enhance Fertility

Achieving work-life balance is critical for people who want to increase their fertility. Workplace stress and pressure can have a substantial impact on both physical and mental well-being, affecting fertility. Individuals can improve their chances of having a child by striking a balance between job and personal life. Here are some tips for achieving work-life balance and increasing fertility:

Make self-care a priority: Take care of yourself physically and mentally. Exercise regularly, eat a well-balanced diet, get adequate sleep, and handle stress. Self-care is critical for improving fertility and general health.

Establish clear limits: Define distinct boundaries between work and personal life. Say no to excessive professional commitments that may interfere with your personal life. Make time for self-care, relaxation, and activities that make you happy.

Time management: Manage your time well to ensure that work-related chores do not interfere with your personal life. To avoid feeling overwhelmed, prioritize and delegate duties whenever possible, and set reasonable goals.

Communication: Keep open lines of communication with your boss and coworkers. Advocate for work-life balance and express any concerns or challenges that may arise. Collaboration and understanding can go a long way toward achieving a satisfactory equilibrium.

5. Use technology wisely: Take advantage of technology. Consider using productivity tools, scheduling software, or apps to help you manage your work and personal life more effectively. Set limits on your technology use outside of work hours to minimize excessive screen time.

Network of support: Surround yourself with a network of family, friends, and coworkers that understand and cherish the necessity of work-life balance. During difficult times, rely on them for support, counsel, and encouragement.

Establish reasonable expectations: Recognize that establishing a work-life balance is a continuous effort. It may not be possible every day, and that's fine. Accept the concept of "good enough" and prioritize progress above perfection.

Workplace flexibility: If possible, look into flexible work alternatives such as working from home, altering your schedule, or negotiating fewer hours. These solutions can provide you with greater freedom and allow you to prioritize your specific demands.

Relaxation practices: To help manage stress, include relaxation techniques in your routine. This can include mindfulness meditation, deep breathing techniques, yoga, or any other activity that allows you to relax and discover inner peace.

Seek professional help if necessary: If work-related stress or fertility issues become unbearable, consult a healthcare practitioner or a therapist. They can offer advice and support throughout your fertility journey.

Remember that striking a work-life balance takes time and effort, but it is critical for improving fertility and overall well-being. You can boost your chances of conception and establish a positive atmosphere for starting or expanding your family by integrating work and personal life harmoniously.

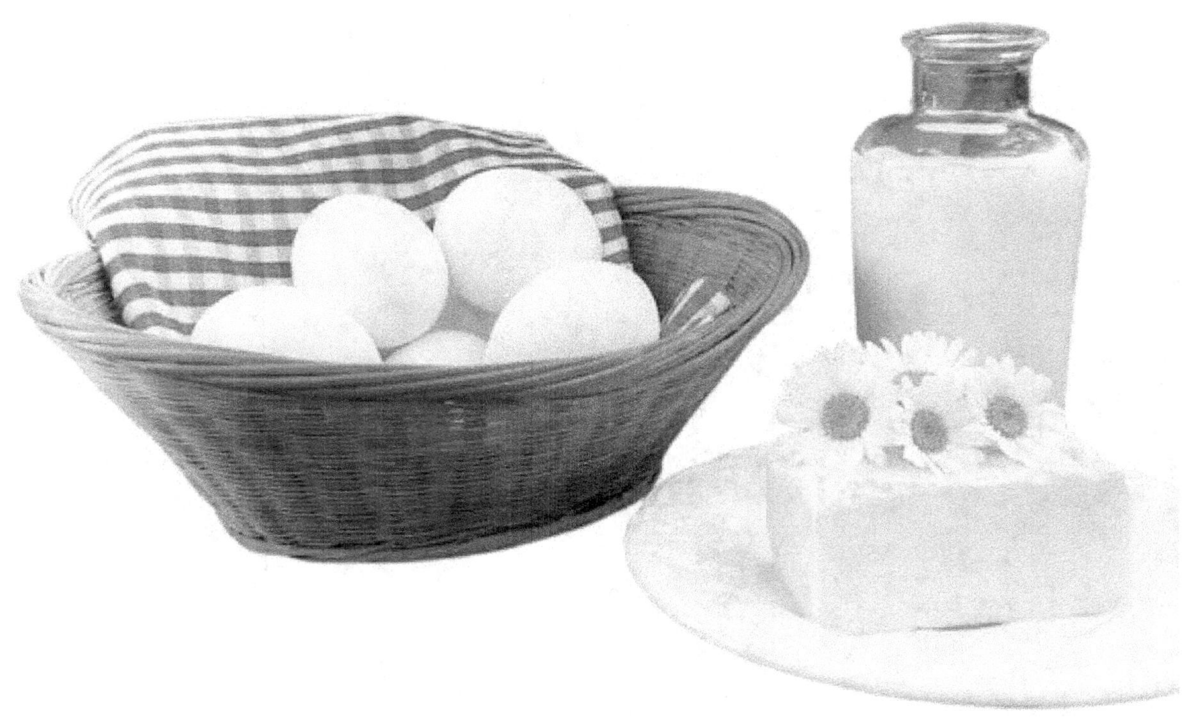

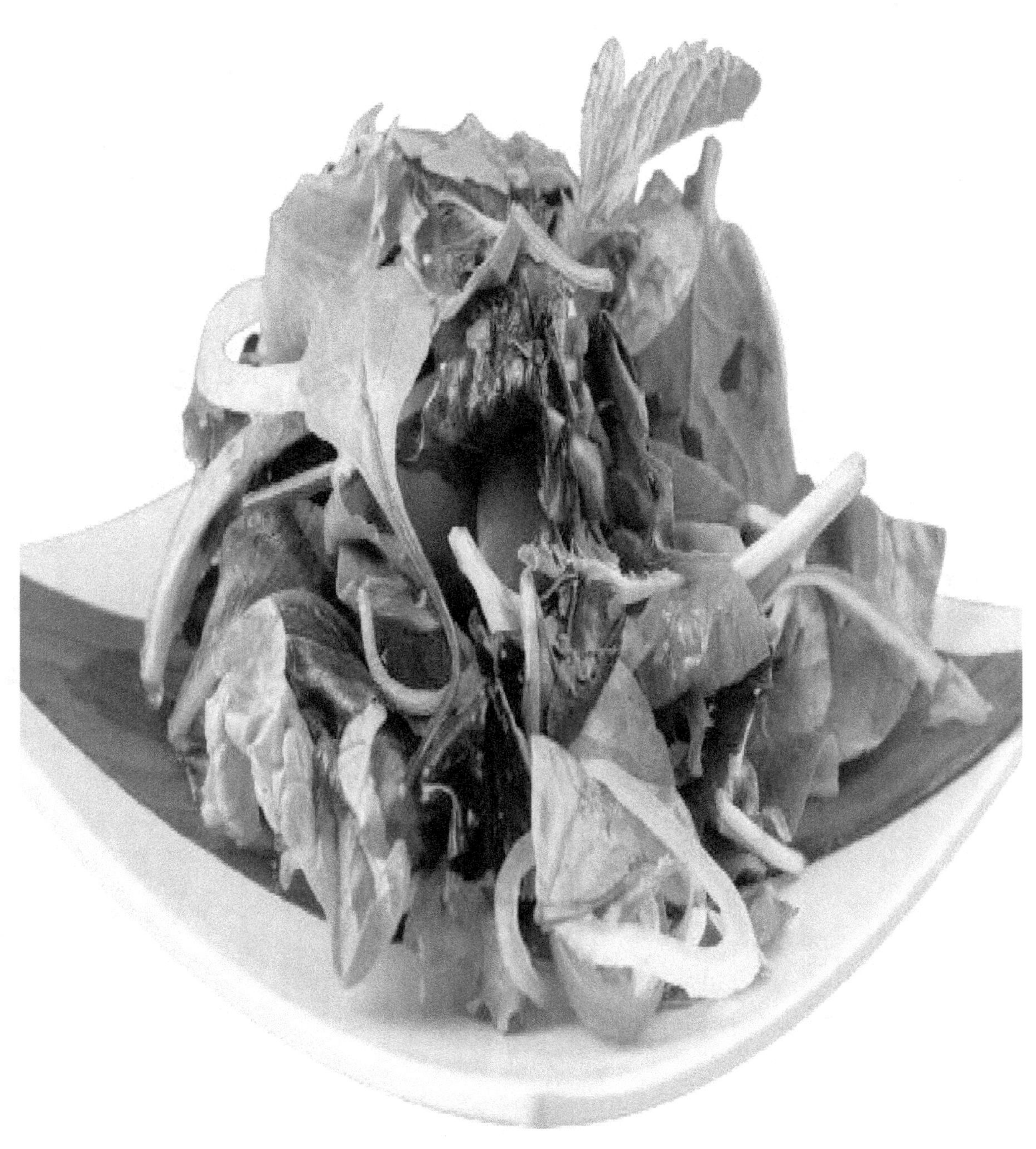

Conclusion

In conclusion, "Fertility Diet Cookbook for Women" is not just another cookbook; it is a comprehensive guide tailored specifically to support and enhance women's fertility journey. Throughout the book, we have explored the significant impact that diet and lifestyle choices can have on reproductive health and fertility.

By delving into the latest scientific research and expert advice, we have uncovered a range of nutrient-rich foods, delicious recipes, and meal plans designed to nourish and optimize fertility. The recipes provided in this cookbook are not only mouthwatering but also thoughtfully structured, taking into consideration key nutrients and their role in promoting hormonal balance, egg quality, and overall reproductive well-being.

Furthermore, the "Fertility Diet Cookbook for Women" goes beyond food to address the importance of managing stress, enhancing sleep quality, maintaining healthy body weight, and engaging in regular exercise - all crucial aspects of maintaining optimal fertility. By implementing these lifestyle choices, readers can significantly enhance their chances of conceiving and achieving a healthy pregnancy.

The focus of this book is not just on women who are actively trying to conceive but also on those who want to prepare their bodies for a future pregnancy. No matter where one is in their fertility journey, this comprehensive guide provides a wealth of information, tips, and recipes to support and enhance reproductive health.

Moreover, "Fertility Diet Cookbook for Women" aims to empower women and help them gain a deeper understanding of their bodies and reproductive systems. By bridging the gap between scientific knowledge and practical advice, readers will be equipped with the tools they need to make informed decisions about their fertility and take active steps to optimize their reproductive health.

It is essential to remember that every individual's fertility journey is unique, and there is no one-size-fits-all solution. However, "Fertility Diet Cookbook for Women" serves as a valuable resource, offering evidence-based information, practical suggestions, and delectable recipes to support women in their pursuit of fertility and overall well-being. By harnessing the power of nutrition and holistic approaches, this book provides a gentle and compassionate companion for anyone looking to enhance their fertility and embrace the possibility of new life.